The Chirurgia
of Roger Frugard

THE CHIRURGIA OF ROGER FRUGARD

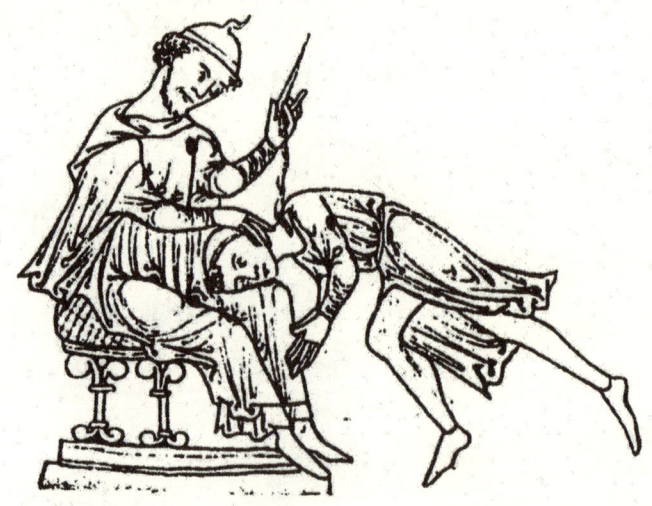

Frontispiece

Surgeon Suturing A Neckwound

From a French Translation of Roger's Chirurgia (1209)
as reproduced from Tony Hunt's The Medieval Surgery
The Boydell Press (Boydell and Brewer, LTD.)
Woodbridge, Suffolk. 1992
p 83

The Chirurgia
of Roger Frugard

Translated from the Latin Venetian
Edition of 1546

by Luigi Stroppiana
and Dario Spallone

Istituto Di Storia Della Medicina
Dell'Universitá Di Roma
Roma 1957

English Translation
by
Leonard D. Rosenman, M.D.

To order additional copies of this book, contact:
Xlibris Corporation
1-888-795-4274
www.Xlibris.com
Orders@Xlibris.com
15064

Contents

BOOK I

THE HEAD

BOOK II

THE NECK, THE NAPE, THE THROAT

BOOK III
THE TORSO FROM THE SHOULDERS
TO THE GROINS
AND UPPER EXTREMITIES

BOOK 1V
THE PELVIS AND LOWER EXTREMITIES

A COMPENDIUM PHARMACOPEIA
OF MEDIEVAL SURGICAL MEDICATIONS

FOR JALJA

Who Keep My Heart

INTRODUCTION

Roger's name first appeared in writing during the last half of the 12th C, when he was recognized as the premier surgeon in Italy. Since then he has been acknowledged as the leading figure in the rebirth of the art and science of Surgery in western Europe, which had been deprived of it for centuries. Yet, is that truly the case?

Who was Roger and whence came he? What were his sources—his recorded practices and teachings certainly were not all new-born in one man? What is his own in the written work which we have only in manuscripts from the hands of copyists? And we know that most of those copies were made after the lifetime of Roger himself; each copy offers us a Roger who was read and copied and glossed according to the lights of the copyist. Most of them were ignorant of the surgical matters contained in the medieval-latin words which they could re-write into many other languages, with little understanding of what the words revealed.

As we sort through the many answers that have been offered during the eight centuries that separate us from Roger, we find few that agree completely in all the points at issue. My own beliefs which follow are a consensus, my assessment of the materials offered.[1]

Roger was the son of an old Parmesan family, and today we call him Roger Frugard of Parma. He may have lived until the end of the 12th or early 13th C. The erudition exhibited in his works indicates some knowledge of the few Latin translations of the Classic and Arabic masters which then were appearing in the Schools. They were the products of the few bookish monks at Salerno and Monte Cassino, especially of Constantine the African and Gerard of Cremona. Because he could read Latin, we assume that he was educated in the classrooms of schools provided by Italian priests and monks at or near Parma. Some of the clerical physicians—a very few of them also practiced surgery—took priestly orders or became monks. The restrictions which prevented the clerical physicians from acting as surgeons were not yet severe in Italy in Roger's epoch, and some of them were married and fathered families, an acceptable practice to some extent even until the time of William and Lanfranchi. However, we have no indication how deeply involved in religious activities was Roger himself during his surgical career.

Where did he learn the rudiments of practical surgery, whatever he could not learn from books ? Did he travel in Italy and Sicily and

---

[1] Who and where?; Baas-Handerson (p.299) say he was Roger of Palermo who became a professor at Salerno, and date his death in 1210. However, Sarton assures us that Roger of Palermo was a translator in the court of Emperor Frederick II, not at all the surgical Roger! And Sarton (Vol II p.439) insists that ours was Roger of Salerno, not Parma. Sarton cites Sudhoff and others to support his view. Garrison (p. 141) calls him Roger of Palermo. Malgaigne (Hamby) says that he was born at Parma and that he was a Salernitan surgeon, but he places him in the 13th C. Corner agrees about Salerno but gives 12thC dates. Nicaise calls him Roger of Salerno who was cited twice by Henri de Mondeville (p xxxv) and once by Guy de Chauliac (p. xlii), and places him active around 1230. DeRenzi was entirely certain that Roger was a Salernitan, but sets his dates later than any body else, ahead by at least a half-century. Daremberg is uncertain of Roger's Salernitan connections. Hunt is adamant in refusing anything except remote contacts between Roger and Salerno. Tabanelli's fascinating explorations in these matters led him to accept a Parmesan birth and to insist on a Salernitan basis for our Master's career. Etc. See bibliog. (LDR).

attend the practices of the unlettered and unskilled and unfettered workers? They had produced a few handbooks, the so-called Practica, in local languages, which are the grim records of the state of ignorance of those times.[2] Their weaknesses set Roger apart from his Italian predecessors and contemporaries; indeed, his book begins the new era. Tabanelli comments that Roger makes little mention of the Classic and Arabic authors who themselves simply cited the works of revered predecessors as proofs for their own claims, that being the 'scientific' method of the times. Tabanelli wisely added, "The lack of citations is not enough to let us accuse Roger of ignorance" (T. p.12). And we have Roger's statement in the Proem to Book I, " I have decided to set down in writing that practice as if it comes from me alone" to explain why he—really via his amenuenses—mentions few 'authorities'.

Early in the 12thC century Salerno was the only place in Italy where some formal medical education was obtainable and where some standards were insisted on. By mid-century Bologna along with Padua, Parma and Naples had accepted some of the translations and personnel and had begun to grow as centers which came to rival Salerno in the 13th C. But Roger had Salerno, and he became its star. As we have noted, Salerno had offered some schooling in Medicine for at least a century before Roger, and had settled on a tradition of excellence which allowed it to grant a sort of license, a permit to practice medicine and surgery. It was a certificate of competence which by 1225 was accepted everywhere in Italy by decree of Emperor Frederick II, and soon in all northern Europe. Only Hunt, among the modern historians, denies a Salernitan schooling for Roger. I am convinced by the

---

[2] Some reference should be made to Calabrian influences. The monastic traditions in that southern corner of Italy included infirmaries and monks who practiced a primitive kind of medicine. Certain religious interdictions inherited from the Arabs deferred the performance of some surgical procedures to Jewish practitioners. The Mss which reveal the extent of the surgery of Calabria and its influences on the Salernitans who followed them in the next century are few and remote. The best modern source is Rombolá, although Pagel (Sudhoff) and Zimmerman-Veith offer some comments on those issues. 0p.cit.(LDR)

weight of evidence that Roger the Parma-born surgeon was a true Salernitan and that his own teaching followed the patterns he adopted from his teachers. *(See footnote 15 at Chapter 19, Book I.)*

For more than seven centuries the surgical treatise attributed to Roger, his Chirurgia, was credited as the first European surgical text, as the product of a Salernitan who later moved to northern cities. However, his book cannot be entirely an 'original', born from him as its sole resource. Roger's feet were planted on the shoulders of predecessors.We find his sources in the translated texts that he encountered at Salerno, and, indeed, in a surgical text of sorts that preceded his own!

That book came to light only in our own century, discovered by K.Sudhoff in the Royal Library at Bamberg. The "Bamberg Surgery", as it is presented in Corner's interesting study, was a loosely arranged collection of materials copied from Paul of Aegina and a few Arabic authors. It was a crude model available to the Salernitans, certainly by mid-century 12, and there is little doubt that Roger used it. The medical historians before the Bamberg History was discovered could not have known of it when they investigated and debated the Rogerine legends.

Now let us trace Roger's career. At some time after he left Salerno he practiced at Parma. His surgical skills and successes and his reputation as a teacher attracted pupils as well as patients. As it was for the seven or eight great surgeons who followed Roger in the next hundred-fifty years, their own disciples requested the treatises which are our only records of the awakening of Surgery in Europe. We know that Roger did not write his own book; it is a product compiled by a group of his pupils and issued sometime between 1170 and 1180, probably at Parma. The editor and leader of the compilers was Guido II of Arezzo. I believe that Roger was alive at the time and that he participated in and approved the work. We know that the book had immediate success at Salerno and elsewhere in Italy where it was reproduced by copyists. Many of those Mss are still to be found in medical libraries through the world, in Latin and in other languages.

Even before the dawn of the 13th C Roger's Chirurgia was the accepted standard text in the Schools. The practical experiences of the surgeons who had used it led them to emend Roger and to provide glosses to supplement what they felt was deficient and to rearrange the order of the materials in Roger's treatise. The added comments were a sort of marginalia which described the later surgeon's own experiences and preferences. Roland Cappelluti whose Chirurgia appeared around 1250 was the first major commentator, and soon after that an interesting book of Glosses was issued which discussed and illuminated the Chirurgia of Roger as it was supplemented by Roland. The Glosses of The Four Salernitan Masters exists today in a very few copies of the original Ms, and it remains a puzzle for curious historians. The long essay by Daremberg which is included in DeRenzi's Collectio is a scholarly debate between two erudite historians and is the best resource on the Glosses. It is an interesting investigation of the Rogerine and Rolandine questions.

The orderly arrangement of the medieval surgical text and the list of its topics were proposed by Roger and modified by Roland, and they were copied with little improvement during the next three and more centuries. The Head to Foot arrangement which was hinted at in Albucasis' Surgery, became the accepted pattern.

Despite its honored traditions in Italy Salerno's dominance of surgical education during the 13th C passed to Bologna and Padua and to other northern cities. The treatises of Bruno of Longoburgo, Theodoric and William of Saliceto became the newer bases for a surgeon's education, and at the end of the century Lanfranchi of Milan carried the lore and the art into France. Yet, without exception, all the authors bowed to Roger in their books. A modern reader of those treatises will see few changes in the accepted surgical treatments, but he will find great differences in the substance of the books by the surgical authors of the ensuing century and half. Roger's terse and sometimes haphazard presentations were replaced and expanded, finally to achieve the rich texture and style of Henri de Mondeville.

For my English translation I have had access to four texts (see bibliography). The Latin Ms of the 13th C which is in DeRenzi's Collectio contains many addenda which have been attributed to Roland. I have included the addenda in my text.[3] There is little to be gained in producing a separate English translation of Roland's Chirurgia. The Italian translation of the Roger-plus-addenda by Stroppiana-Spallone comes from that Latin Ms. It is the immediate source for most of my work. Tabanelli follows Stroppiana for his own Italian edition, taking the portions he uses with almost no changes. However, as he did in his edition of Bruno, he eliminates many parts of the text in order to provide a compendium of abbreviated medieval surgical treatises for the Italian reader. Tabanelli's insertions are interesting, challenging and informative asides, valuable for any serious reader. I am much in debt to him.

In addition to the three Mss above, I have used Hunt's edition of Roger. It is an Anglo-Norman translation which appeared in England at the close of the 13th C. The copyists produced a text which is different from the Latin in many ways. The chapters are broken apart and the topics are renumbered. Many prescriptions differ as to contents and dosages and methods of preparation. Nevertheless, we can see that the surgeon of Norman England had in hand a treatise very much like his contemporary's in Salerno or in Bologna. I owe much to Prof. Hunt for his meticulous historical and linguistic investigations of Roger and for his illustrated texts. I am grateful for his encouragement.

---

[3] DeRenzi's edition (Vol.II p. 425) cites the editor of the Venetian edition of 1546 as evidence for the attribution of the Addenda to Roland. In his edition of Roland which accompanies that of Roger, Tabanelli states (p 123) "...we maintain that Roland 'captured' the work of Roger, simply adding the fruits of his own experience."(LDR).

ACKNOWLEDGMENT.

I offer my sincere thanks to the Librarians at the Harris Fishbon Memorial Library at Mount Zion Hospital/UCSF, for their patient efforts in my behalf.

This English translation is a product of the Department of Surgery at The Mount Zion Hospital of The University of California in San Francisco, encouraged and supported by the Chairman, Professor Orlo H. Clark. Also, I am deeply indebted to the Mount Zion Health Fund for assistance in obtaining the publication of this book.

BIBLIOGRAPHY

Albucasis. On Surgery and Instruments. transl. by Ms Spink and GL
Lewis. Univ. of California Press, Berkeley. 1973. The Surgery is the
last of Albucasis' grand medical compendium of thirty treatises
published just before or after 1000.

Baas, JH. Outlines of the History of Medicine, Transl. and supplemented by HE Handerson. reprinted by Krieger Publishing Co.,
Inc. Huntington, NY, 1971. Original German edition of 1889

Bruno of Longoburgo. see Tabanelli

Capparoni, Pietro. Magistri Salernitani Nondum Cogniti. John Bale,
Sons & Danielsson. London. 1923

Corner, George. On Early Salernitan Surgery And Especially The
"Bamberg Surgery". Bulletin of the Inst. of the Hist. of Medicine.
Vol V., pp. 1-33, jan., 1937

Corner, George. The Rise Of Medicine At Salerno In The Twelfth
Century. Annals of Medical Hist. New Series Vol III, pp. 1-16, Jan.
1931

Daremberg, Charles. Introduction To The Glosses Of The Four
Salernitan Masters. in S. De Renzi's Collectio Salernitana, Vol. III,
pp. 205-254.

De Renzi, Salvatore. Collectio Salernitana in five volumes. Forno
Editore, Bologna, 1853. Vol..II contains the Venetian Edition
(1546) of a13thC Ms of ROGER, pp.425-496.

Garrison, Fielding. History of Medicine, Third Edition. WB Saunders Company, Philadelpia, 1921

Guy de Chauliac. See Nicaise

Hamby, Wallace. Surgery and Ambroise Paré. Translated from the French of Malgaigne. University of Oklahoma Press, Norman, 1965

Henri de Mondeville. See Nicaise

Hunt, Tony. Roger's Chirurgie. In Anglo-Norman Medicine, Vol. I., pp. 3-138. DS Brewer, Cambridge (UK) 1994.

Lanfranchi of Milan. The Science of Surgery (1295). From a Middle-English Ms. of 1380. Edited by Robert von Fleischhacker. Early English Text Society. London, 1894. Engl. transl. by LD Rosenman. l999. Awaiting publication

Malgaigne,JF. See Hamby

Nicaise, E. Guy de Chauliac's Grand Chirurgie, 1363; edited and translated by EN. Germer, Balliere et Cie, Paris, 1890

Nicaise, E. Henri de Mondeville's Chirurgie,1306-1320; edited and French transl. by EN. Germer, Balliere et Cie, Paris, 1893. Engl. transl. by LD Rosenman, 1998, awaiting publication

Pagel, JL. Einführung in die Geschichte der Medizin (2nd Ed. by Sudhoff). S.Karger. Berlin, 1915. pp. 169-170.

Roger. See De Renzi, see Hunt, see Stroppiano, see Tabanelli.

Rombolá, Franco. Storia della Chirurgia in Calabria (V-XX secole). Edizioni Emme Elle, ed. Eugenio Santelli. Mendicino. 1989. pp 7-31

Rosenman, LD. A Medieval Surgical Pharmacopeia, 1999. Awaiting publication

Sarton, George. Introduction to the History of Science. Williams and Wilkins Company, Baltimore. Three Vol. 1927-1948.

Stroppiana, Luigi and Spallone, Dario. Ruggiero da Parma, CHIRURGIA. Istituto Di Storia Della Medicina Della Universita Di Roma. Rome. 1957

Tabanelli, Mario. An Italian Surgeon of the Thirteenth Century, Bruno of Longoburgo. Leo. S Olschki, Florence. 1970. Engl. Transl. by LD Rosenman awaiting publication.

Tabanelli, Mario. La Chirurgia Italiana Nell'Alto Medioevo. Ruggiero (pp.x-105 ff) Ruggiero-Rolando-Theodorico. Leo S Olschki, Firenze. 1965.

Theodoric Of Bologna. The Surgery. edited and English transl. by E.Cambbell and J. Colton.. Appleton-Century-Crofts, Inc. Two vol. 1955 and 1960.

William of Saliceto. Chirurgie. edited and French Transl. by P. Pifteau. Imprimerie Saint-Cyprien, Toulouse.1898. Engl. transl. by LD Rosenman, 1997. awaiting publication.

Zimmerman, LM and I Veith. Great Ideas in the History of Surgery. Williams and Wilkins Company, Baltimore, 1961. p.94.

A NOTE ABOUT THE TEXT

Roger's Chirurgia contained four Books and an introductory Proem. The 'head-to-foot' arrangement controls the contents without special concerns for order according to types of lesions or diseases, although trauma receives the greatest emphasis.[4] Book I deals with the head, Book II with the neck, Book III with the torso and Book IV with the arms and legs. Unlike Roger, later authors arranged their treatises with head-to-foot displays of their materials in separate Books, according to the nature of the disorders : wounds, fractures, other diseases, etc. Daremberg's essay includes a discussion and examples of that change.

Roger did not provide a separate Book devoted to Cautery or an Antidotary. Therefore, I have prepared a Compendium Pharmacopeia as an appendix. It lists and briefly identifies all the simples and a few of the compounds used by Roger and the other famous surgeons during the century and a half after him. I have culled the seven great surgical treatises written during that epoch. Roger's list is recovered in large part from Hunt's edition of the Anglo-Norman Ms, in which he provides an excellent glossary. The Roger-Roland Latin Ms and the Italian translation of Stroppiana include a rich resource of remedies in the many Addenda attributed to Roland Cappelluti. Therefore, this Compendium includes some, if not all, of the substances used by Roland other than those he found in Roger's text.

Each remedy in the Pharmacopeia and Formulary is marked with

---

[4] Tabanelli comments (p.20) that this should be understood to be a product of the war-filled times which occupied Europe, especially the Mediterranean countries. (LDR)

the initials of one or more authors who mentioned it. Those cited for Roger are marked **R**. In the text itself, I have used modern vernacular names for plants and metallic substances where that is feasible. Other matters identifying the medications can be found in the Pharmacopeia.

Each of the four Books in Roger's Ms was preceded by a list of the chapters by name. I have placed those lists in a Table of Contents which opens this translation.

A NOTE ON STYLE

Roger's text as it appears in the Ms printed in De Renzi's Collectio and as translated by Stroppiana-Spallone will be translated in plain face type. My own parenthetical insertions in the text will be identifed by (ie). Insertions taken from the other Mss and comments relevant to the text will be printed in Italic-face, and identified by H if by Hunt, by T if by Tabanelli, by D if by Daremberg and by R-R if taken from the Roger-Roland Ms in DeRenzi. The sources of footnotes will be identified in parentheses, by LDR if by me, and by the others' initials.

BOOK I

THE HEAD

PROEM

After the creation of the world and all of its contents [5], God wished to create Man from the clay itself and to instil in him a vital spirit of almost heavenly quality. As I say, he took a mean and fragile matter to add weight to a celestial substance of a sublime and marvelous consistency, resembling the Creator Himself, to be preserved by his grace on a par with the celestial beings.[6] From the very beginning material Man would be part of the Earth; with his second endowment he would be clasped in the Lord's embrace, so long as he continued his proper observances (ie of The Lord's precepts).

In God's wisdom he first formed Man without defects; he endowed him with a free will and he explicitly prescribed what he should do and what he must avoid.

Because he violated the Divine precepts, Man brought upon himself various punishments, assigned to the various parts of his makeup. He went from certain knowledge to a state of ignorance. From a regency over his own domain he became an exile. Where once was light now were shadows. Where he had found delight he found misery, going from joy to sadness. In all cases, based on His fulsome justice, sadness replaced its opposite.

The Supreme Physician reserved for himself the treatment of the spiritual parts and to us physicians he relegated the treatment of the

---

[5] This opening phrase was used frequently rather than the simple title to identify Roger's treatise (LDR).

[6] The soul had angelic properties (LDR).

body's ailments. Our treatments of the latter have a theoretical basis and we administer them accordingly.

So it is, in the human body various disorders have internal or external causes. This Treatise deals with the benefits of treatments for each, by setting forth the interventions proper to each case, giving each method its own label.

The practical measures, then, are remedies for the corruptions caused by external agents and by openings in the body (ie wounds), and we provide similar benefits by uniting what has been opened.Those activities are what comprise Surgery.

After a plea that I could not deny, from my Colleagues (ie his disciples) as well as other illustrious persons (ie the physicians), I, after a full discussion and deliberation, have decided to set down in writing that practice, as if it comes from me alone. My ambition is this: whoever will have used these treatments as handed down from me will pass them on, whereas I, for my part, can retain everlasting honor and fame.

I have realized, for some time, that the work should be divided into parts which deal more specifically with the different parts of the body, in order to more reliably prescribe treatments and to carry them through to the desired results. Take note (ie of the advantage of the arrangement): When a diligent surgeon has been able to diagnose accurately an illness and can localize it to any of the four parts of the body by seeking out the signs and symptoms, he will be able to use the appropriate treatment (ie to find it in my book).

Now let us go first to treatments for ailments of the head, it being the most noble part of the body, proceeding from the head as a whole to its individual parts.

Book I has forty-four Chapters. I have placed Roger's rubrics in the Table of Contents

CHAPTER 1.
WOUNDS OF THE HEAD

The head may suffer various sorts of injuries, with or without fractures of the cranium. At times a fracture may be large and easily detected. But, large or small, the accompaning wounds (ie of the soft tissues) may be large and gaping or small simple incisions.

Whenever the cranium is broken we must ascertain if the membranes of the brain are damaged, either the pia mater or the dura mater. The signs of injury to the latter are : headache, a flushed face, wide-open eyes, blackened tongue.

The signs of injury of the pia mater are: general feebleness, loss of voice, pustules on the face, discharge of blood from the nostrils and ears, constipated bowels.

(R-R or diarrhea which is even more serious), and shaking chills three or four times a day, which foretell a fatal outcome. Furthermore, most of the above signs predict death before one hundred days. When the damage in the meninges is extensive, death will ensue at the time of the next full moon.

Although all fractures of the cranium present serious threats, we should diagnose them with care and try ro intervene as best we can.

Addenda by Roland

A. Note that when constipation or diarrhea ensue, the risk is indeed serious that the outcome will be fatal.

B. Another bad sign: is the extremities lose their natural warmth, right to the tips to the toes.

C. The effects of the celestial bodies are noted, especially that of the moon, on the accumulation of fluid: when the moon enlarges the accumulation of fluid in the affected part increases, especially the increase of fluid in the brain, which emits froth which it cannot contain. If the brain cannot vent the fluid the patient will die.

Chapter 2.
Displaced Fractures With Open Wounds

When the fracture is obvious and the wound is large and open, such as made by a sword or the like, you first should remove the loose bone and other foreign matter. Remove the fragments immediately unless the hemorrhage is too brisk. Use a quill and carefully insert a piece of thin soft cloth almost all of the way between the dura mater and the fragment .[7] Then, [8] lay a linen or, even better, a silk cloth into the opening, large enough so the edges of the cloth can be tucked under the peripheral margin of the intact cranium, to prevent the discharges from the open wound from contaminating the dura mater and threatening harm to the underlying brain.

Then continue to wipe the wound dry of the accumulating pus, using a clean and dry sea sponge, as you would use blotting paper. Fill the mopped wound with pieces of linen which you have soaked in egg-whites and then squeezed almost dry. Lay a pad on top of the

---

[7] A delicate maneuver to detach the loose bone fragment from the underlying dura mater (LDR).

[8] Here the surgeon treats a fracture freed of loose fragments or perhaps one with a simple separation at a linear fracture (LDR).

wound and the surrounding region and carefully wrap and tie a bandage. Change the dressing twice daily during the winter and thrice in summer time *(H: Because during the summer months wounds make more pus)*. Have the patient lie with the wounded side down *(H: to favor drainage away from the dura)* Continue this regimen faithfully until the fracture has united.

Addenda by Roland.

A. Unless the depressed bone is removed promptly a syncope will occur. *(H: Sometimes the surgeon will not be called to attend a patient until days after the injury and the wound already is suppurating. In such cases the fragments of bone etc. must be removed at once.)*
B. Silk is better because its surface is less abrasive.
C. Use a quill or splinter of bone to insert the cloth.
D. The sponge must be thoroughly washed to rid it of the salts which will corrode the dura mater. All astringent substances are hot, and corrosives are hot as well as dry.

CHAPTER 3. PROUD FLESH
(GRANULATION TISSUE) ON THE DURA MATER

When foul or necrotic tissue delays the healing of the fracture and covers the dura mater use a well-washed and dried sea-sponge placed in the wound to keep the overgrowth dry. After the bones have been united (ie by callus), treat the proud flesh itself with a powder of hermadactyl. Dress the wound with shredded linen or cotton, so-called charpie. After the bones are bound together securely, use the Apostles' Ointment , which contains 1/2 lb. of black naval tar, 1/2 lb; serapinum, armoniac, and opoponax, 1/2 ounce each; wax, 3 ounces.; and wine vinegar, 1/2 lb.[9]

The Formula for The Apostolicon

Put some vinegar into a tin bowl and add the resins which have not been ground beforehand, that is, the galbanum, armoniac, serapinum, opoponax and the black tar. Then add the wax while heating to melt all. Then add a little cold water until the mix has a proper thickness and its color changes. Then add the Greek tar which you have ground into powder. Also add the mastic and the olibanum in equal amounts. Stir and mix continuously until the color is a pale yellow. Remove the pot from the flame and add and gently stir in the terebinth. Pour all into a linen sac which will filter the material that is squeezed out and add some oil of laurel or similar and rewarm the mixture as you stir until you can see the water in it boil. Then form it into madeleines (ie rounded patties).

This surgical apostolicon also is good for treating the spleen (ie a 'medical' disease). After the bones are bonded anoint the wound. The ointment works both for the healing of the bone and the wound. It relieves the pain of fractured ribs, caused by contusions.

---

[9] This is the first of several warnings not to use ointments and oils when they can find their way to damage the meninges (LDR).

Addenda by Roland

A This powder (hermodactyl) is mildly corrosive.

B. The charpie is combed and scraped from cloth.

C. Use more wax in the summer than winter because of the melting effects of heat, and less in winter to lessen the hardness of the ointment.

D. We use a tin vessel here because it is a cool metal for use in melting ointments and syrups. We use bronze, a warm metal in vessels for oxymel and plasters.

E. Some surgeons disapprove of the drying and erosive effects of the apostolicon.,

CHAPTER. 4 CRANIAL FRACTURES WITH SMALL (NARROW) SCALP WOUNDS

When the fracture is large and the wound at the surface is small you may find it impossible to assess the full extent of the fracture. In that event insert a finger and by touch examine the fracture thoroughly to learn what you need to know. There is no better way. After you determine reasonably accurately the dimensions of the fracture, use your sharp razor to make a criss-cross incision and lift the scalp from the surface of the bone with a scraper. Delay that if the fracture bleeds too freely or another complication appears *(T: perhaps syncope).* Then (ie if the hemorrhage is not a problem) use a forceps to remove bony fragments and other foreign material.

However, if the bleeding is excessive, defer the maneuver until it stops. At the first opportunity act quickly to remove the undesirable things. Then, with great care, insert a cloth tent between the dura mater and the bone and follow that with the dressings we have described heretofore. Bring together the edges of the incision and fill the gaps in the wound with strips of linen which you have soaked in egg-white and wrung out. Apply a pad over all and bandage it. Leave on the dressing until nightfall, or over night (ie if the first dressing was applied in the evening). Edema of the corner flaps is a good sign, but if the flaps are shriveled and retracted, that bodes ill. Persist with your treatments until the bones are healed. Reduce the volume of linen or charpie packs and allow the flaps of the cruciate incision to fall together as the healing progresses.

In cases where we have determined that there is a fracture we do not bathe the wound until the second or third day and then we insert as a drain a cloth moistened with egg-white only and we never introduce an oily substance. Use the apostolicon only on the surface of the skin when we can be certain that is away from the wound edges.[10]

Change the dressings and bathe the wound no less than two or three times a day. Do not introduce any oily substances. At the very end of the process you may use some apostolicon on the skin.

This is how I make another ointment for my own use. You may use it safely around (ie not in) the wound. Place some saffron in water and let it stand until the water is well colored. Filter it and add wheaten flour and mix well while bringing it to a boil. Keep it for use. It will mitigate and soothe the pain.

Addenda by Roland

A. Probing with a quill or metal instrument is less sensitive (ie than the finger).

B. Urgent treatment will avoid syncope.

C.and D. Re the four corners: Place a linen pad over the base of each 'tail' pressing inward, and a tampon over the tips, so to prevent reentry of pus beneath the flaps.

E. and F. The edema indicates that the nature can provide nutrition; the shriveling indicates a blockage of the vital substances.

G. The initial application (ie in the case of a fracture) is an irrigation of egg-white (ie before insertion of the drain).

---

[10] The apostolicon could leak through the fracture line and offend the dura mater (LDR).

H. The early appearance of pus is a good sign; a late appearance is
   bad. As Hippocrates stated, a dry wound is bad. Soft matter is
   good, hard is bad.

Chapter 5. Linear Cranial Fractures

In the case of an undisplaced fracture where one fragment does
not ride below the other, one may not be able to tell if the fracture
goes all the way through to the brain. To demonstrate it have the
patient pinch his nostrils and close his mouth while he exhales
strongly. If something *(H: fumes)* appears through the crack you will
know that a fracture is full-thickness. In that event do this:

No matter the length of the fracture-line, if nothing stands in your
way (ie hemorrhage, etc.), use a metal trephine and carefully drill
holes on one or another side of the fracture-line, making as many
openings as you will need. Then saw *(H: chisel)* from one hole to the
other along the entire fracture line. That will create an opening
through which you may remove the pus which has accumulated on
the surface of the brain (ie on the dura). Tuck a cotton-wool or fine
linen cloth between the bone and the brain with a quill, the full
length of the defect.

Then treat the wound with our usual methods.

Addenda by Roland

A. When inserting the saw (ie the elevator) in the fracture line take
   care not to injure the dura mater.If the fracture is not so large as to
   involve the brain (ie to cause symptoms), use a rasp to scrape away
   some bone at the fracture and remove enough to expose within to
   determine whether or not the fracture went full-thickness through
   the cranium.

   (*H: When one side of the fracture is partly depressed and the fragment is
   easily separated from the intact cranium, remove it and treat the remaining soft-
   tissue wound and fracture as you learned above, with the saw and all the rest.*)

CHAPTER 6. HEAD-WOUNDS WITHOUT CRANIAL FRACTURES

When the head-wound is only in soft tissues, simply and carefully bring together the wound edges with a cloth dressing soaked in egg-white and wrung almost dry.

In winter times use a plaster until the wound suppurates, which I make as follows: Take malva which grows in gardens or other types and some branca ursina, dock, pellitory and convolvulus. Crush them and mix them thoroughly with a half pound of lard. Then put all in an earthenware bowl and add two or three ounces of wheaten flour, two ounces of flaxseed and two ounces of fenugreek and some white wine. Mix again and set the bowl over a low flame and stir with a spatula until it thickens. Then set it aside to cool before use. Another good maturative: equal parts of honey and wild celery and some flour.

In summers: Take some leaves of nightshade with three ounces of malve and grind them in a mortar with three ounces of unsalted veal-fat. Then take some more solatrum and yellow-horn poppy which is called wild celandine. If you have no celandine use pennywort, and take some cassilago, henbane and violet herb. Grind them all and remove the liquid *(Hunt's copyist adds: "to which you add an equal amount of wine ")* and mix in three ounces of wheaten flour and three ounces of fresh honey. Stir it over a low flame for a long time until it arrives at the proper consistency. Then set it aside (ie for use as needed).

Another poultice for application in different seasons (ie the Black Ointment described below) is spread on a piece of linen cloth and used until the wounds suppurate. When pus appears use dry packs until the wound dries. Then replace the cloth with fluffy charpie. When granulation tissue proliferates remove all the packings, strips and fluff. But from the time of first suppuration, as noted above, until the wound is dry, use only the Black Ointment (ie on the strips and charpie) which we make as follows:

Take one pound each of ordinary (ie olive) oil and mutton fat, five pounds of naval pitch and three ounces of greek tar. In summer time take three ounces of wax, but use only two in the winter. In summers take two ounces of mastic, and five ounces each olibanum, armoniac, galbanum, serapinum, opoponax and terebinth. Put the oil, the black tar and the gummy simples in a pewter pan (ie they have not been ground with the galbanum, armoniac, serapinum and opoponax) and place it on the stove. Grind the mastic, olibanum and greek tar together (ie while the others are heating). When the pan's contents are melted add the ground up substances while stirring with a spatula. You will know when the recipe is ready when a droplet place on a marble tile sticks to your finger and is not easy to peel off. Then remove the pan from the fire and add the terebinth (ie which loses its potency when heated) and strain all the mixture through a cloth. Set it aside. This ointment is very good for use in all fresh wounds. It induces the formation of healthy granulation tissue and scar.

The remainder of the treatment is according to our protocol.

Addenda by Roland

A. Do not stir egg-whites too much. They will lose their freshness.
B. The reference to leaves is for the althea (malva).
C. The first plaster above is called the surgeon's mush.
D. In another book of this treatise red wine is used. I quote, "after adding pure red wine, heat it.."
E. For relief of pain after the contusions apply a paste of honey, wine, cinnamon and oil. If the plaster is not effective against pleuritic pain, you should bleed the patient.
F. Use the black ointment as soon as pus appears.
G. Be aware that the temperature of the simples in the compounds affects the wound: warmth invigorates the part. Cold constricts the openings from the veins and causes retention of the fumes and vital spirit, thereby potentiating the natural heat. Warm and moist elements, such as fenugreek and linseed, potentiate one's natural heat and their moisture wets the matter in the wound (ie it loosens the crusts, etc.). That is an added value.

The cold substances of themselves by constricting the outflow from veins and arteries retain the fumosity of the vital spirits, and reinforce the natural warmth as they promote maturation (ie suppuration)). Note that a plaster made with elder-tree sap and fine millet flour is good for relief of pain and chronic swelling.

CHAPTER 7. SWELLINGS OF THE HEAD CAUSED BY BLOWS

A blow may cause a swelling on the head and yet make no open wound; there may or may not be a fracture beneath it. In the former event the fracture may not be evident and the edges of the fracture may not the palpable. However, when you can feel the displaced bones you should proceed to make your cruciate incision and do all the other things for treating cranial fractures.

Addendum by Roland

A. In such injuries treat with phlebotomy before the blood in the contusion can coagulate, and immediately apply astringents. If the contusion is not fresh, use diaphoretics and maturatives.

CHAPTER 8. WHEN A CONTUSION CAUSES A HIDDEN FRACTURE

When the fracture simply is a crack (ie not palpable) make your diagnosis by these clinical signs which you should be able to recognize. By the fifth to seventh day after the injury the patient cannot eat or drink (ie nausea) and his digestion is bad; he is sleepless; his urine and feces are scanty and he is feverish. By these signs you will know that there is a fractured skull which you will treat with incision of the scalp, etc.[11]

---

[11] Whatever were Roger's sources for these chapters on Head-Wounds, we know that very much of what he wrote was already available in the Salernitan school. The socalled "Bamberg Surgery", much of which was directly copied from the Pantegni of Haly Abbas and Paul of Aegina, provided sections which are found almost verbatim in Roger's Chirurgia. See *Salernitan Surgery and the Bamberg Surgery*, G.W. Corner; p.18 (LDR).

Addendum by Roland

A. In these cases the scalp may be lacerated. When the cut exposes the cranium you should free the skin from the bone and suture it. Then sprinkle on the red powder. Follow with the treatments already described. Be aware of the need to repair the muscular layers as well as the skin, as we explained in the chapter on that subject.

CHAPTER 9. CONTUSIONS WITH SWELLING IN THE ABSENCE OF SKULL FRACTURES

In such cases the diagnostic signs of the previous chapter are absent. Therefore, you treat only the swelling with the following poultice:

Take some absinthe, vinegar, artemisia, wild celery, onions, rue and cumin. Grind them, add oil and bring to a boil. Place the mixture over the swelling and renew it two, three, four or more times a day, as hot as the patient will tolerate. If that plaster fails to cure the lump, change to this one: Take a fistful each of absinthe, artemisia and common malva and grind them. Add three ounces of lard and four of wheaten flour and mix them with some wine and place it all over a flame while you stir with a spatula until it thickens. Use it as a poultice on the swelling until it comes to a head or is absorbed. If the former, incise it with an instrument called a sagittella and express the pus with your fingers. Then treat the wound as if it were a carbuncle or other abscess.

Addendum by Roland

A. Before using the plaster, try astringents such as solathrum and sempervivum. Then apply diaphoretics, and at the end, use maturatives if the others fail. Diaphoretics usually are the most successful.

CHAPTER 10. A SCALP-WOUND WITH CRANIAL INVOLVEMENT

When a blunt object (a stone, etc) causes an open wound in the scalp and creates a dangling flap under which the bone is seen to be fractured, you remove the fragments by trepanation. Then you suture and attach the flap to the intact scalp using a square (ie cutting-edge) needle with a silk thread. Insert the needle through the flap first, and take bites spaced about the width of a finger-nail apart, to apply the edges of the wound to fit each other nicely.

At the lower end leave a gap through which you may treat (ie medicate) the underlying wound. Atop the surface apply our consolidative red powder, made as follows: Take one ounce each of consolida (ie consoude) major and bol d'armenie, three ounces of greek tar, one half ounce each of mastic and olibanum and two drams of sangdragon. Mix all and grind carefully. The powder serves to control hemorrhage and as a consolidative for bone and for soft tissues after the suturing of the skin over them. Atop the powder lay a leaf of broom or similar. We usually insert a tampon and a pad over it at the end of the wound to collect the discharges and to allow easy access for our medications.[12]

If the surgeon has made an incision (ie to treat the fracture) we insert a cloth strip wet with egg-white, and go on the treat that wound with our usual medications as we described for cranial fractures.

The suture powder should be dusted on two or three times daily for nine days, or until you see granulation tissue coming through the gaps between the sutures, from within the united parts. Then you should cut the stitches at skin level and judiciously ease them out over time. Cover the wound with a linen dressing or the like until it is completely healed.

Addenda by Roland

A. Dried and powdered human blood has therapeutic value, like mummy, which it can subsitute for.

---

[12] Note the implication that the external application of the topical medicine - here it is a powder - has effects in the deeper tissues (LDR).

B. If the leaf which you lay on the wound is a consolidative it will have the same effect as any other consolidative. The same holds if it is a corrosive, or a maturative, being effective as if it were such a drug.

Chapter 11. Open Cranial Wounds With Fractures

If the incised scalp wound enters the bone and is such that you can reach and treat and remove fragments of bone from beneath the scalp treat the wound as we have described. If not large enough you must operate as you now know how.

If some scalp has been cut away (ie by the weapon), exposing an intact cranium, treat as described for such wounds.

Addendum by Roland

A. In the latter case you can use the Yellow Ointment, an oily substance, without concern that it will penetrate and harm the dura mater.[13]

Chapter 12. Wounds of the Scalp On The Dome Of The Head

An open wound, anterior or posterior, which is deep enough to injure the brain is mortal. However, even it extends the length of the scalp. even to the ears or to the nose, but does not affect the brain, it is not lethal. Treat it as you would any other wound.

Addenda by Roland

A. These wounds lie over the junctures of the cranial commissures.
B. If you encounter subcutaneous swellings (ie such as wens, cut into by the wound), grind flaura[14] and artemisia and moisten them with rose-water and egg-white, and use as a plaster.

---

[13] Because the cranium is intact (LDR).

[14] The herb flaura probably was a leafy aristolochium or fumitory (LDR).

CHAPTER 13. ON SUTURING WOUNDS OF THE FACE.

When the face, that is, the nose, the lips and other important and delicate structures of the body, are cut, they should be repaired by suturing. First approximate the edges as accurately as you can and then sew only the outer skin. Use interrupted sutures placed with a sharp needle armed with silk thread. The intervals between stitches should be small.

If it so happens that the nose and lips are wounded by the same stroke, fit the parts together as neatly as you can and sew them. Then lay pads alongside the nose and hold them in place with a bandage that resembles a horse's halter to keep the parts in proper alignment. You may have to insert a drain in the nostrils to provide a channel for the escape of pus or for irrigations. Leave a gap at the end of the wound to allow pus to drain freely and also to allow you to insert a drain. But when the bones are cartilaginous as in the nose or ears or penis (ie compressable by the external pads) you must not block the canals with internal packs.

Use our red powder on the surface for nine days and follow the instructions to the letter.

Addenda by Roland

A. A running suture is better.
B. If you don't have our red powder, use bolo armenico or pulverize some flakes of oven-soot, or some charred great mullein or broom, together or separately, or use powdered frankincense or mastic.

CHAPTER 14. ARROW-WOUNDS OF THE FACE.

If an arrow strikes the nose, near the eyes, the cheeks or else-where on the face and the metal arrowhead goes deep or enters hidden recesses or follows an irregular path, the process of extraction may be difficult. Nevertheless, each case requires its own clever solution and plan of attack. If some of the shaft remains in the wound it may be attached to the metal. Slip a strip of cloth into the full depth of the wound alongside the shaft (ie to act as a guide), the track being short. If the wood and metal remain firmly attached you can gently rock them bit by bit and pull on them very gently and you may be able to remove them.

But if the metal tip is detached, learn from the patient just how he was wounded: in what position he was when he was struck, from above or below, from the front or the side? Then insert a probe into the wound of entry and try to determine the path created by the arrowhead, to find it and to remove it. If you cannot do that without harm to the patient, leave it alone. Many people have lived well with metal in them.

If you do extract it, immediately introduce a strip of bacon (ie as a drain). If it does not reach the bottom, make a tent of linen smeared with pork fat and push it in. Dress the wound with cloth compresses. Bandage from the bottom up, so that pus can be expressed. Healing will be delayed by a collection deep in the wound and favored by drainage from the bottom.

Use this dressing and bandage until pus no longer appears in the opening (ie the arrow-wound may be only a small perforation in the skin) and keep it open as long as it takes to avoid trapping pus being deep inside. That dictum holds for all wounds.

If you want to induce suppuration, in addition to the different drains inserted in the wound use plasters—differing in winters and summers—as we described in earlier chapters.

Use various items to suit the case. But, do not allow the wound to become dry (ie scab over). Withdraw the drains (ie shorten them) only as the wound is cleansed (ie from the depth).

CHAPTER 15. WOUNDS CAUSED BY BARBED ARROWS

In such cases do this: Try to introduce a dilating forceps and carefully grasp the metal head and remove it by following the track of the wound. Failing that insert a slim metal tube, iron or bronze, to reach one barb and to slip over it; then go to the next barb. With great concentration and patience you can extract the arrowhead. You may use a hollow goose-quill instead of a metal tube. Follow with the usual treatment for wounds.

CHAPTER 16. OTHER WOUNDS OF THE HEAD

The upper part of the head (ie above the hair-line) may not be in the usual line of flight of an arrow or the like and the treatment for that kind of piercing wound may be difficult but not beyond hope.

When an arrow or other weapon penetrates the skull through and through—from front to back or the reverse—follow these rules: If there are no presenting signs which forebode certain death, immediately incise the scalp at the wound of exit and drain the cranium through a trepanation, shaped as a letter C if possible (ie not just a drilled hole). Make it large enough to enable you to remove the arrowhead easily. If some of the shaft remains, you may be able to remove the weapon through the wound of entry.

For others, if the arrowhead does not go all the way through the cranium and if good signs prevail through five to seven days, make your incision near where the tip or a bit of shaft can be seen, as we describe (ie cruciate), and enlarge the hole in the bone using a sharp trephine. After detaching loose pieces, remove the the arrow. The rest of the treatment is as for fractured skulls.

Addenda by Roland

A. The lethal signs which appear when the dura or pia mater are injured may not be due to a tear but may be caused pressure from the arrow spear.

B. However, do not make a C-shaped trepanation, but make it to extend along the bone from the wound of entry to the wound of exit, following the track of the of the shaft of the arrow between the bone and the dura mater. Make a fissure in the bone, as well as an incision in the fleshy tissue of the scalp.

C. The bad signs which may appear three, four or five days after an extraction of an arrow are due to damage to the dura mater. Those signs forebode death and have been described: anorexia, insomnia,, fever, etc.

CHAPTER 17 ON DEPRESSED FRACTURES WHEN THE SCALP IS INTACT

When the bone is depressed by a blunt force which does not open the scalp, the brain's functions may be somewhat impaired *(H: because the bone presses on the brain)*, as when the patient has nightmares of himself in combat with an enemy and he awakens from sleep and siezes his own weapons and acts as if he is wide-awake.

The treatment includes a cruciforn incision in the scalp, elevating the scalp with a rasp, perforating the bone by trepanation and elevating the depressed bone. The treatment then follows the methods already described, especially those at the beginning of this section on head-trauma.

CHAPTER 18. TINEA OF THE SCALP

One can distinguish curable from incurable tinea of the scalp by these signs. In incurable cases the skin is thick and hard and the tinea produces a lot of crusts and it eats away the hair. We leave those hopeless cases untreated.

Curable tineas appear in one of two ways. In one the hairs are plentiful and some may be bristly, and the scalp is thick but it is not broken and it is not indurated. In the other the skin is thick and fissured and it itches badly, and it may ooze pus. You treat both types with the same measures.

First shave the head. Then apply this ointment: Take one ounce each of white hellebore and naval tar and six ounces of walnuts. Grind all together and make an ointment. In winters you may add some walnut oil to the above to thin it. Rub the ointment into the scalp—about one ounce for each of nine days, or longer as you find the need. When the skin recovers depilate it by pulling out the hair by the roots and apply more ointment liberally, every day. When the hairs grow back wash the scalp with lye. When the scalp is dry apply a silotrum (ie a depilatory) and leave it on until the hairs come away easily. Make it as follows: Put four ounces of quick-lime into a pot of boiling water. After a long boil add one-fourth ounce of arsenic (ie yellow oxide of) to the water as it boils. When it has boiled sufficiently, a feather dipped in the pot will lose its tufts as they fall from the quill. Apply it to the scalp and the skin will redden. Repeat the above routine until the redness and swelling are gone. If that fails, use this ointment: Take one ounce each of staphisagra seeds and white hellebore: five ounces each of arsenic, vitriol and alum, and one ounce of oak gall. Mix and grind to a powder and then add seven ounces of olive oil-dregs (faex). Then add a handful[15] each of clover-leaves (ie herb flaura) fumitory and domestic and wild artemisia, wild mustard, titimalle (spurge) and dock. Mix all and grind out the the juice which you mix with the oil-dregs and set to boil. Then add back the ground up residue from above and add three ounces of liquid resin (ie probably turpentine). Use this as an inunction on the scalp and continue with the treatments described for the other ointment.

If also there are many lice use an ointment of quicksilver tempered with saliva. Afterward you may treat the rough healed skin with lard followed by resin and the silotrum used above.

---

[15] Handful". A misleading term. The Latin maniple and the Anglo-Norman javele are not precise. The amount may vary from a large man's fistful to a dainty lady's 'pinch'. The reader must assume that a pinch of a spice or of salt will suit a prescription where other ingredients are measured in drams and ounces, and that a handful of leafy stuff will be suited to several pounds of lard or oil, etc.

A splendid discussion of weights, measures and dosimetry in medieval pharmacopeias is included in T. Hunt's *Popular Medicine in 13thC England*, 1990, D.S. Brewer, Cambridge. pp 59-63 (LDR).

If the tinea is of recent (less than one year) origin and not yet chronic, we need not depilate: simply treat as follows: Another ointment: Take a handful of artemisia, fumitory and wild mustard. Grind together and steep in oil for three to nine days or more as you see fit. Bring to a boil. Apply as hot as the patient will tolerate, morning and evening. Then dust this powder on the lesions: Grind equal parts of staphisagra and white hellebore, and use it freely until the cure is complete.

Addenda By Roland

A. A complete cure is indicated by a white skin and normal hair-roots.
B. For lice: Smear a woolen thread—or even better of a silk—with attenuated mercury and tie it around the head. The lice will adhere to the thread and can be eliminated. However, attenuate the mercury with saliva and ashes of human hair.
C. Dust the staphisagre powder between the hairs (ie on the fissured skin).

CHAPTER 19. ON SWELLINGS (SUPERFLUIDITIES) ON THE SCALP (IE SCABIES)

Some swellings on the scalp are called ruva or rufa in the Salernitan dialect[16], and we treat it (scabies) with this ointment: Take two ounces of live sulfur, one ounce of white hellebore, one of quicksilver, and five ounces each of cumin and gutta percha.[17] Mix and add six ounces of soft lard to make an ointment to rub on the head It is the recommended treatment. You may try this same ointment when treating sores on the face (salt phlegm) and painful lesions on the legs the legs.[18]

---

[16] Tabanelli calls attention to this remark as a certain indication of the Salernitan origin of Roger or at least of a close follower. The R-R Ms (about 1250) states " quae vulgari salernitano ruva seu rufa dicitur" (LDR).

[17] Gutta percha probably was staphisagre, socalled caput purgium (LDR).

[18] I assume that Roger here refers to various crusted ulcerations on the face such as acne or even basal-cell cancers, and to venous stasis ulcerations on the legs (LDR).

Addendum by Roland

A. This ointment is useful for gangrene and all sorts of ulcers. But it produces dryness of the lesions and much suffering thereby, and I do not approve of its use. I avoid it in the young and delicate patients since the treatment itself can increase the risk of death.

CHAPTER 20. OTHER SWELLINGS ON THE HEAD

Some of the swellings resemble scrofulas; one type is firm and the other is soft. The first is movable whereas the other is fixed. Treat the mobile one (ie sebaceous cyst) by grasping and lifting it and holding firmly with your fingernails while you incise along its axis and dissect out the contents with the intact membrane, using a spatula. If you cannot remove the membrane (ie the cyst lining) fill the cavity with a cloth pack wet with egg-white. After a day replace it with a powder of asphodels which will corrode and destroy the membrane; make it so. Take six ounces of asphodel juice and three of quicklime and one ounce of arsenic. Mix well and boil the fluid and the lime while stirring in the arsenic. Reduce to near dry and set in the sun until you can form the damp powder into trochés for storage. This powder will eat away and cure the mass. When you see that the tumor is swollen and dry, apply a cloth wet with egg-white and lay atop it a stupe of oakum with whole egg. Wait until the membrane rots and the wound has a little pus. Then treat it as you did head wounds without fractures.

In a case of a fixed mass make a cruciate incision over it and scrape out the contents. That will allow you to inspect inside and to remove the membrane. When you cannot remove the sac the turtle (ie sebaceous cyst) will tend to recur.

Another kind of fixed mass is a scrofula which penetrates the scalp and the cranium and seems to arise from both. Some seem to arise from the dura mater itself, but really, the scrofula usually takes origin from the bone.[19]. The treatment includes removing the overly-

---

[19] Tabanelli suggests that this penetrating scrofula is the 'talpinaria' described by Lanfranchi, Yperman and Guy de Chauliac. He cannot identify it in modern terms, although certainly Guy's description suggests an abscess with osteomyelitis. Guy follows Roger very closely! (LDR).

ing (ie ulcerated) skin, trephining all around the diseased bone and elevating it from the dura with a spatula in order to remove it in toto. Cutting the disease from the dura mater (ie where it even may be rooted) is a perilous undertaking. I advise that you do not do it.

Addenda by Roland

A. The mass is called a testudo (turtle), because it is shaped like a boss. As noted, the movable ones can be cured by making a cruciate incision and scraping out the contents. Then get rid of the lining membrane. Failing that, the mass will recur. Note, also, that some of the testudos may take the shape of chestnuts.
B. Be aware that the arsenic loses its potency when it is heated.
C. Use the asphodel powder for five to seven days .
D. That kind of immobile scrofula (ie adherent to the dura) is not curable.

CHAPTER 21 THE TREATMENT OF MANIA AND MELANCHOLIA

In cases of mania and melancholia we make a cruciate incision at the crown of the scalp and we perforate the cranium to allow the escape of the offensive matter (ie vapors) while the patient is restrained by bonds. Then we treat the wound with our usual methods. In cases of epilepsy we burn at the nape of the neck in the hollow beneath the tip of the occiput.[20]

CHAPTER 22. OCULAR DISORDERS

At times the eyes pour out tears and become red and lid-hairs turn inward. That causes a burning irritation as well as lacrimation. At times those symptoms appear without abnormalities of the eyelid-hairs. When the eyelids are abnormal, treat the patient as we will describe in the following chapters.

---

[20] Hunt's Ms, Chapter 26b, states that the purpose of the cauterization is to produce drainage of pus (LDR)

CHAPTER 23. DISEASES OF THE EYELASHES

If the eyelashes are abnormal (ie probably ectropion) and there is proud flesh which covers the lashes, first rub the lower lid with leaves of pellitory until the granulations bleed and shrink and you can see the hairs. Then pull them out by the roots using a tweezer. Then lay on a lot of egg-white. In the winter add a little saffron and repeat the operation as new hairs appear. Bind the lids shut with some pressure. When there is less proud flesh again rub the lids as above until they bleed and continue the treatment until all the matter is gone. Then take the juices of blackberry twigs, absinthe and egg-white and apply it over the lids.

CHAPTER 24. LACRIMATION WITH RED EYES

When the tears overflow and the eyes redden in cases where there are no abnormal eyelid-hairs, bleed the patient from veins on the forehead and from two places on the temples. After what you deem to be a sufficient amount, lift the pierced vein with a threaded needle, with care not to perforate the vein. Repeat the passage of the thread and doubly ligate the vein to prevent any further bleeding. Dress that wound site with lard for three days and then go to salt-pork strips changed daily for ten days. That will leave a clean wound when you remove the thread and get rid of the local granulation tissue. If necessary apply a pad of charpie or the like.

To reduce the lacrimation, pierce the hollow of the cartilage of the ear with a seton.

Another treatment: anoint the temples and the wound-site with this: grind olibanum, frankincense, mastic and labdanum, in a heated marble bowl and add a leaf of laurel. Apply it as hot as is tolerable on the veins in the temple, noted above.

Chapter 25. Itching Eyes

To eliminate itching use a collyrium made as follows: Take five ounces of litharge, one-quarter ounce each of olibanum and hepatic aloes. Grind them to a powder and mix with some oil of violets, or use juice of wild celandine, one or the other, achieving the consistency of a white ointment Introduce it as a collyrium into the eyes with a hollow quill. If burning and smarting persist use this collyrium: Make a powder of litharge, hepatic aloes and mastic. Then take some buds of blackberry and some wormwood twigs in equal amounts and squeeze out the liquid. Add it to some rose-water. Then mix in the powder. Drip it into the eye.

Addendum by Roland

A. In the last prescription, if you have no rose-water you may substitute rain water, juice of broom, or of polygonum, or of dogwood. Then add the wild herb. The quarter-part dose of wild herb and aloes is tolerated in the eye; apply it externally as well as within. Labdanum is very irritating. It is better to insert the seton in the hollow beneath the ear. Even better is the application of a nodular cautery tip (ie at that site).

Chapter 26. On Cloudy Films In The Eyes
(ie Conjunctivitis)

To eliminate the films over the eyes I usually apply this ointment. Take a handful of darnel (salvia) and celandine and crush them with a pestle. Add six ounces of common oil and allow to sit for five to nine days or longer until the leaves shrivel. Then boil until the herbs settle at the bottom. Remove from the fire and strain the liquid through a cloth. Replace over the flame and add one ounce of wax and melt.

Then test by putting a drop on a marble tile where it should adhere. If so, add two ounces of flower of brass (ie or verdigris) and slowly bring to a boil. Again test with a drop on the tile. If it has a green color, remove it from the flame and add two drams of olibanum and mix in two drams of powdered spode. Then add two drams of powdered sarcocolla. Finally add six drams each of honeysuckle and hepatic aloes. Add more oil to thin the mixture while stirring with a spatula. When it has been thoroughly blended, strain it and keep it for later use.

Use a hollow quill to drip it into the corners of the eyes. When the film is gone, take rue and scarlet pimpernel and the juice of an earthworm, the so-called pectina, mixed with oil and apply it in the eye. The worm is good for other blemishes, too.

Another good powder for the same purpose: Take two drams each of beaver-musk, olibanum, sarcocolla and five of camphor; two drams of intact pearls (undrilled); one dram of bronze flower. Grind the musk and olibanum and some frankincense and the verdigris in a clean warm marble bowl. Stir all until they are dry and grind with a pestle until finely powdered. Powder the other ingredients separately, including the pearls. Then combine the powders in a clay pot and mix in some rose-water Then rub them through a cloth sieve before moistening with more rose-water in the earthenware bowl. Set it in the sun to dry for three days before adding more rose-water. Repeat the cycle of drying and moistening three times. After nine days all the ingredients will be a shrunken dry mass., and may be kept until you need it it. As a powder it will clear the membranes from the eyes.

Addenda by Roland

A. Concerning spode; it is very effective in this ailment as it has corrosive powers.
B. Sarcocolla either is the juice of an alien (ie overseas) herb, or, according to others, of the camomille family. If you have none, use celandine in its place.

C. The powder described last, above, is used when the itching is bad.

CHAPTER 27. REDDENED EYES

When the eye is red due to blood or other cause for swelling or films, bleed from veins on the forehead. After shaving the areas, have the patient place his palm *(H: at the wrist)* at the base his nose with his fingers spread, laying out a pattern resembling a halter. Use ink to mark where the tip of the fingers touch the scalp and where the outstretched thumb touches the forehead (ie temple), three fingerbreadths above each ear. Connect the marks with ink-lines and incise the skin along the marked lines (ie to cut the underlying veins) and allow the wounds to bleed *(H: to drain pus!)*. Then apply a hot cautery along the incisions.If the patient is feeble and will not tolerate that maneuver, make the marks as above but incise along only one line. Cauterize and treat the wounds with pads moistened with egg-white and other medicines to mitigate the pain and calm the patient. Bandage the head as you did for other wounds and leave the burn-wounds open for thirty to forty days. After removing the bandages allow the wounds to close.

CHAPTER 28. BLEEDING IN THE EYE AFTER A BLOW AND OTHER CAUSES FOR SWELLING

When such occurs, do this: Take fresh wax and add powdered cumin and melt carefully to make a plaster. Apply it warm. It is a good remedy.

Another treatment uses vervain and absinthe. Squeeze out their juices and mix with rose-water and make compresses of oakum or similar. In winters add some safron because that also is very effective.

Addendum by Roland

A. White absinthe mixed with rose-water is a good remedy. If it doesn't work at first, repeat the application three times. Remember that for ocular problems we use resolutives followed first by decongestants and finally by diaphoretics.

CHAPTER 29. A SCAR OF THE EYELID AS THE RESULT OF INJURY OR INFECTION[21]

If a crease (ie inversion) forms in the lower lid the result of an abscess in the lower lid or the bad result (ie scar contracture) of an old wound, make an incision to drain pus and to accept a perforated (with four holes) lead plate which you suture to the upper edge. Lay a small pad on the center and bandage it to press it upward. Leave it for nine to eleven days before you remove the lead plate. Then treat the wound as we recommend.

CHAPTER 30. FISTULA NEAR THE EYE

Occasionally a fistula forms near the eye and drains purulent matter through a tiny opening. In that case push in an instrument to dilate the opening or cut it open to accept a strip of cloth wet with egg-white inserted to the very bottom. If the patient is a delicate type, place a slim bronze tube into the already dilated tract, if possible, to the bottom. You thread a hot iron (ie wire) cautery through it to burn the roots of the fistula. If the patient dreads the hot cautery, introduce through the cannula a bead of corrosive ointment made from potash-lye and quick-lime (ie 'a virtual cautery'). Leave it there from the third to the ninth canonical hours or from the nones to the vespers. Then insert strips of cloth with egg-white, repeated until the

---

[21] The substance of the text suggests that the Ms use of "inversion" does not mean entropion, rather that the outward rolling of the lower lid was caused by a contracting scar which pulled the edge downward and everted it. The crease was the 'inversion'. Roger incised transversely, parallel with the scar, sutured the lead disc and applied pressure upward to eliminate the contracture (LDR)

inflammation subsides and the medication is gone. Then simply treat the wound. Make the ointment by adding the lime to the lye and mix it well and make a simple salve (ie added wax).[22]

Addendum by Roland

A. To make the potash-lye take two parts of burnt beans (ie ashes) and one part of quick lime and grind them to a powder. Spread the powder evenly at the bottom of a small basket and compress it by treading on it in the basket after sprinkling it with water. Spread more powder, add more water and build it layer by layer to fill the basket. Then burrow a narrow hole about six inches (ie one-half a cubit) deep with a kitchen-knife. Place a tub under the basket and fill the hole with water three times a day. Collect what drips through during the first eight days. Test its potency by suspending an egg on a string in the lye. A strong lye will reject the egg.

CHAPTER 31. FLESHY EXCRESCENCES IN THE NOSE

Sometimes the superfluous tissue is a polyp, sometimes it is of another type. At times it remains intranasal and at other times it may extrude to reach the lip. Treat a polyp thus:

Lift it gently with a spatula to expose the base. Then cut it off with a curved knife. The after-care varies: If some tissue remains near the nostrils you may use one of several corrosives based on quick-lime and soap, followed by egg-yolk in olive oil. If inflammation recurs, use our methods for treating inflamed wounds with green ointment, etc.

Prepare Green Ointment as follows: Take handfuls each of celandine, oxalis (leaves and roots), salvia, wild lovage and scabious. Grind them with a pound each of ram's tallow and oil, and let it sit for nine or seven days. Then heat it in a tin pan until the herbs sink to the

---

[22] Note the admonition to use this method for delicate patients. In the alternative treatment, advocated by the classic authors, the hot wire was pushed through the nasal bone into the nose itself! (LDR).

bottom. Sieve it and reheat the product as you add three ounces of wax in summer or two in winter. After the wax melts add five ounces each of powdered olibanum, mastic and verdigris. Test the consistency of the ointment before and after this last addition and observe if it turns green. When that happens remove it from the fire and add five ounces of powdered hepatic aloes. Remix it with oil (ie to achieve an ointment) and save it for use.

You may use the green ointment for chronic plague (ie ulcers); it regenerates healthy tissue after it has destroyed the bad.

If the proud flesh appears in the nostrils (ie not as a pedunulated polyp) and obstructs them insert heated strips of ciclamen, repeated two or three times if necessary to restore the nasal passages before using the green ointment.

Chapter 32. Nasal Polyps

A true polyp appears within the nose and sometimes grows larger in the rear and obstructs the airway and dilates the passages as it enlarges. Some polyps are incurable. the signs are a dark and indurated nose, a blackened polyp whose base is not edematous. The nose is soft in cases of curable po;yps and can be maneuvered to allow us to cut and cauterize. Grasp the polyp delicately with a tenaculum and draw it out of the nostril where you can extirpate it. Failing that, simply cut off as much as is exposed. If even that is not possible, dilate the nostril with a tampon containing dry ciclamen and then insert a hollow metal tube through which you place your cautery and burn off the polyp. Then apply egg-yolk in oil until the ensuing inflammation subsides. Then use our standard wound-care.

When a patient rejects the feared actual cautery, inert a strip of cloth (ie probably through the tube) containing a corrosive. Then use the egg-yolk, etc.

Sometimes the polyp appears behind the palate.That is the result of its natural enlargement. Treated it by excision. Then use waxed tampons in the nose until healthy epithelium appears. In such cases, cauterize the forehead using the three-fingered pattern described in the chapter on ocular inflammations. Be extremely careful to cauterize only as deep as the scalp muscles and not to reach the cranium. The rest of the treatment is as described.

Addenda by Roland

A. The polyps often are caused by catarrh which descends (ie from the cranial cavity) to the nose where it accumulates. Treat that by purging the excessive humors. If the cause is a cold humor use laxative pills containing castoreum or pigra. Follow the purge with doses of yellow olibanum. This same order of treatment is to be used for gangrene and fistulas; that is, always precede the local measures with purges. Finally, note that polyps usually are caused by cold humors and rarely by hot, which become cool after the purges.

B. Do not apply the cautery suddenly or with heavy pressure. Avoid damaging the brain with excessive heat.

CHAPTER 33. CANCERS OF THE NOSTRILS[23]

Cancers appear in the nostrils as well as in the lips, palates and gums. The affected tissues are eroded and sometimes reddened (ie inflamed). The swollen skin is not eroded but the cancer corrodes inward.[24]

When the flesh of the lesion is hard and purplish black the cancer is difficult to cure. You will find it easier to treat less ulcerated lesions of recent origin in this manner. Cut away the cancer with a razor until you reach living tissue. Then apply a hot cautery.

Follow that with applications of whole eggs and oil until the burn reaction subsides. If any of the cancer remains, apply a corrosive ointment and follow with the eggs.

---

[23] The terms 'cancer' and gangrene' were interchangeable long after Roger's epoch. The differences between ulcerated neoplasms on exposed surfaces and ischemic necrosis were not fully recognized (LDR).

[24] A fair description of the rodent ulceration of basal-cell carcinoma (LDR).

When a cancer invades the lip or nostrils and has corroded some of the structures, cut it away and treat as above.

When the gums are involved (ie probably pyorrhea rather than neoplasm) wash them with vinegar and alum for three days before going on to this liquid: Take equal parts of boiled wine and honey-vinegar and boil it with great mullein, honeysuckle, pomegranate peels, pyrethrum and ginger. Apply by rubbing the gums until the lesion is dry.[25] Then use this powder: equal parts of alum, rose petals, oregano, pomegranate peel, roasted date pits, pyrethrum, cinnamon, nutmeg and aloes. Grind all to make a powder. After using it, wash the region with hot vinegar and apply calamint. You may have the patient chew wild lovage leaves. After the gums are clean, keep the left-over powder in a sac.

Another good remedy: cloves, cinnamon, date pits, olive leaves, alum, and leaves of lovage. Make a powder to use after the vinegar and wine irrigations.

Addenda by Roland

A. These cures are not always possible.

B. Avoid excision and cautery in vascular and nerve-bearing regions.

---

[25] The term 'dry' meant free of pus. The surgeon used what were called mondificants (ie detergents, exsiccatives etc.) to cleanse a wound of the pus which he himself had promoted with his maturatives. When creamy pus appeared early, or had replaced foul, pink or gray pus, he then sought means to 'dry' the wound, to favor the agglutination of the surfaces which were lubricated by the pus. He recognized the infectious nature of spongy granulation tissue which oozed pus and delayed the healing . The pyorrhea described here belonged in that category and was treated to make it 'dry'.

The appearance of creamy and not malodorous pus, therefore, was a desirable phenomenon, because it represented a non-corrosive and non-necrotizing discharge from healthy pink surfaces. Hence it was 'laudable'. The fact that uncontaminated fresh wounds will heal without pus and the delays caused by seeking and treating it, was the most significant contribution of medieval surgery. It was promoted by Hugh of Lucca and passed on to Theodoric and to Henri de Mondeville. However, the reaction to that idea by the hide-bound surgical and medical establishments of northern Italy and all of the rest of Europe was a rejection which lasted during more than six hundred years of abysmal folly (LDR).

C. The gums may be puffy and bleed easily and produce foul breath. They may shed their teeth. They seem to be invaded by pus and are not really fleshy. Use the powders described above.

D. Here is he best powder to use after the cancer is excised and after you have used the (corrosive) powder of asphodels; also, it best for drying, eating away bad flesh and regenerating the healthy: Take handfuls of myrtle leaves, domestic and wild salvia, saxifrage and calamint. Dry all, and make a powder of them and apply.

CHAPTER 34. SPLIT LIPS

In Italy they are called setole (ie rhagades). We treat them as follows: Take some henbane and put it on some charcoal embers covered by a funnel. The affected patient should suck in some of the fumes that come through the neck of the funnel.

Another treatment: take equal amounts of hepatic aloes, litharge, vitriol and olibanum and make a fine powder. Then squeeze the juicy from some fumitory leaves and mix it with the powder. Add oil of lard or olive oil, either one or the other, each in full measure. Medicate the lip.

Addendum by Roland

A. Heat some walnut shells to derive the oil. Put it in the split lip. It works wonderfully.

CHAPTER 35. BURNS AND BITES (PUNCTURES) OF THE LIPS

For burns use alum mixed with a little honey. Add that to the ointment in the last chapter and use it on the lesion.

For bites: take flour and sugar and add the syrup (ie honey-alum).) and use it to allay the pain. Or you may use the white ointment made with rose-water instead of vinegar and with oil of violets instead of olive oil.

Chapter 36. Dislocation Of The Mandible

When the heads of the mandible are dislocated from their joints the signs are: the lower teeth do not jibe with the uppers, they are held apart downward or are retracted and the patient cannot move his jaw or chew.

Treat it this way: Grasp the angles of the mandible below the ears and bring the jaw forward into a postion where the dentition of both jaws meet. Take care in that maneuver (ie not to go too far). Then bind the jaw to lift it from below. Apply an oil of althea or the Soldier's Ointment (ie the Martiaton). Be sure the 'bite' is accurate, fitting the lower molars against the upper, and allowing no movement of the jaw. Alimentation is limited to what needs no chewing.

Chapter 37. Fractures Of The Mandible

When the mandible is broken the surgeon can feel the site of the fracture and he can replace (ie by palpation) the fragments to their proper alignment. Keep in mind the contents of the previous chapter on mandibular dislocations. The bandaging, the topicals and the diet will be same here.

If the soft tissues are lacerated in addition to the fracture, first set the bones and then use your best skills to carefully suture the wound, as we described for lacerations of the nose. Leave unsutured an opening at the lower end of the wound and place a drain to fit that opening. Dust our red powder over the suture-line, as we have taught.

Place pads (ie as splints) under and over the mandible and wrap the bandage as each case requires. Change it two or three times a day, according to the season. We have mentioned the diet previously.

Addenda by Roland

A. Suture only those wounds which are large enough to need it and if the wound-edges do not come together nicely (ie without sutures) to form a scar which will not be an ugly contracture. Even in sutured wounds the scar may be deforming when the edges of the wound do not match. All surgeons who suture facial wounds must do so with care to avoid that outcome, that is, to a avoid contracture or an overlapping final scar.

B. The pads should be wet with egg-white. Place a large pad with a central opening over them. The perforated pads are useful in treating all wounds because they allow the surgeon to clean the wound, to apply his topicals and to rebandage without disturbing the underlying dressings.

Keep the dressings in place for eight or nine days until the fracture is secured (ie by callus). Then you can cut the bindings and remove the inner pads. Then apply astringent plasters over the fracture-site.

Chapter 38. Fistulas From The Jaw

When fistulas drain from the jaws some have small openings, others large. Treat the first by inserting a cloth drain containing ciclamen (ie in a powder of the dried tubers) to dilate the opening. When it is large enough, introduce a corrosive ointment to soften and eat away (ie the scarred lining of the tract). That accomplished, follow with drains wet with egg-white to allay the inflammation. Then introduce green ointment or similar, just as we treat other kinds of wounds. Search diligently to determine if the bone itself is the source of the drainage (ie osteomyelitis of the mandible) as after a dental abscess.

When thick white pus appears, the fistula is soft. When the drainage is thin and watery, be concerned that the source is in the roots of a tooth. Treat that simply with a drain covered with green ointment. Follow with the rest of our treatments.

In the mouth use the powders we approved for treating inflamed gums (pyorrhea).

Addenda by Roland

A. The (ie diseased) bone at the root of a fistula must be removed with a scraper or saw before the soft tissues of the fistula can heal.

B. The discharge from the fistula can tell you what humor is at fault. You must identify it in order to use the correct medicine. You can recognize watery phlegm (ie saliva) as white and thin. If it is yellow it is bilious (ie choleric). If dark or black it is cancerous (ie melancholic).

CHAPTER 39. TOOTHACHE

We apply a hot cautery to the hollow behind the lobe of the ear when treating painful teeth and gums.[26] Then we place a (ie medicated) tampon on the cavity in the tooth. An additional measure uses equal amounts of henbane and garlic heated over embers of charcoal, covered by a funnel. The patient draws off the fumes from the vent into his mouth. Those fumes are a wonderful and reliable mitigant of the pain.[27]

---

[26] The Cautery as a surgical instrument had three types of functions. The one most familiar to us was to char, coagulate and destroy tissues which will slough away as eschars and leave behind a clean granulating surface. That function included hemostasis by charring blood vessels and the blood iteslf. A substitute for the hot metallic instrument (the 'actual' cautery) for some uses was a corrosive and coagulative topical medicine the 'virtual' cautery).

A second function did not destroy tissue except to produce tiny burns in the skin over edematous regions and arthritic joints, which acted as counterirritants to produce mild local inflammation and the comforts of local warmth. The third function was akin to that of acupuncture where a pointed cautery or one with a tiny rounded tip was applied in various regions to specifically affect disorders in other parts. The mystique and the benefits were very much like those of acupuncture. Schemes of 'points' were differently favored by the authorities. The mystique included the choice of the shapes and the sizes of the cauteries and a system for measuring the appropriate temperatures according to the color of the heated metal. Various metals had special qualities; the use of gold wires was favored for this function by most of the writers. Other factors influenced the techniques, including astrological phenomena (LDR).

[27] Henbane was one of the substances in the famous soporific sponge which the ancient and the medieval surgeons used as an analgesic (LDR).

Addendum by Roland

A worm can cause a toothache, as we can infer from the cavity in the tooth The treatment includes applying a cautery directly on the affected tooth. If that fails, extract the tooth if it is loose. However, the extraction of a solidly rooted (ie not moveable) tooth is risky, and that includes breaking the tooth and activating humors, even injuring the brain.[28] For such cases use honey boiled in an egg-shell, applied hot.

In cases where the bad humor (ie the cause for the toothache) descends from within the cranium or arises from the stomach, you must not use a cautery until after a good general purge.

CHAPTER 40. PUSTULES WHICH APPEAR ON THE FACE

Treat facial acne and pox as follows. Mix six ounces of frothy honey with two ounces each of the milky sap of figs and the juice of ciclamen tubers. Put the mixture in a scooped out half of a ciclamen tuber and place it over a charcoal grill to bring it to a boil. Add the powder made from one ounce each of white pepper and sugar-alum, two drams of borax and two ounces each of olibanum and squid bones. After grinding and mixing the solids with the liquid save it for use.

Reheat it before applying it on an open sore. When the crust over a pustule splits open apply the ointment there. However, instead of vinegar use rose-water, and use oil of violets instead of olive oil.[29]

Make the White Ointment so: Use five ounces each of mastic and olibanum; one ounce each of litharge and burnt lead; three ounces of white lead. Grind them to a powder in a mortar and add some vinegar and then some oil, bit-by-bit as you stir. When the ointment is smooth and spreads evenly, the topical is ready. It has many other uses: against salty phlegm, for treating the pustules and scabies on the face which are caused by that phlegm, against corrupt humors and impetigos and for relieving dryness of the mouth.

---

[28] This commentator recognized the serious consequences of a retained root in a dental abscess which goes on to osteomyelitis, sinusitis, etc. (LDR).

[29] This misplaced sentence is a copyist's error. It belongs in the next paragraph. (LDR).

CHAPTER 41. SWELLINGS OF THE FACE

There are many such lesions, among them are impetigo, serpigo and morphea, all of which may appear elsewhere on the body.[30] Inasmuch as they are more conspicuous on the face we will deal with them here.

For impetigos we do this: Place some wheaten flour on a blacksmith's anvil and press it with a red hot plate. Apply bits of the hot extruded oil on the lesions. The salty phlegmatic defects also respond to this treatment.

Another topical, useful for lesions of serpigo [31] : Take tartar from white wine, yellow lead oxide, ciclamen juice, a roasted melon, powdered pyrethrum and olive oil. Mix all while adding ciclamen juice and oil alternately. When it is blended keep it for use as needed. Apply it in suitable cases and leave it in place for three days. Then you may wash the face. Repeat as necessary until cured.

Addendum by Roland

A. I prefer a mixture of soap and ground tufa (ie bol d'armenie) smeared on the lesions. Or I use soap and yellow arsenic or soap alone. The juice of celandine is best for chronic (years old) spots on the eyes.

CHAPTER 42. WHITE MORPHEA (VITILIGO)

White morphea can be cured but not the black. You can diagnose the curable type by pricking it with a needle; it will bleed. The black

---

[30] These old terms are loosely defined. Impetigos were pustules with some erythema; serpigo probably included psoriasis and some basal-cell carcinomas; morphea included some cutaneous leprous lesions as well as vitiligo of any sort. Salty phlegms were areas of puffiness, perhaps beneath the eyelids or over an aching tooth, as well as acne vulg. and rosacea, all ascribed to accumulations of salty humors. The humor was classed as 'against nature' and was called 'false'. I think that the similarities of the written 's' and 'f' misled many copyists, and led to confusions of terms in the treatises (LDR).

[31] Here Stroppiana erred. He wrote impetigos where the Latin Ms used serpigos (LDR).

type will leak only white water (ie edema). Use this ointment for the curable ones: Take tartar, live sulfur, yellow arsenic, incinerated salt, crystal salt and soap. Take quicksilver, myrrh, litharge, white wax, oil of beaver musk, laurel oil, goose fat, pepper, mastic, olibanum and calamite (storax). Grind these last-named and combine them with the others, adding the sulfur and the soap and the oil last. Bring it all to a boil and strain it through a cloth. Take some more of the wax and goose grease and mix them with the laurel oil. Only after these are well blended do you add the first-named above. Use the ointment hot, applied twice daily.

Another useful remedy contains equal amounts of stick-sulfur, yellow arsenic, burnt salt, soot, eyes of pike-fish and oil. Grind all and boil. Anoint repeatedly.

And yet another: Take three ounces each of live sulfur, saracene soap, French soap and ground walnuts; two ounces each of tartar and soot; one ounce each of yellow arsenic, common salt and white helle-bore; five ounces of alum; a pinch of fumitory and lapis lazuli and some juice of flaura. Grind all solids to a powder and add the liquid. Mix at length until the blend is smooth. This ointment also is useful against impetigo.

Another for the same: Take roots of asphodel, yellow arsenic, quick-silver, litharge and oil. Grind the solids to extract the liquids from the roots and mix them. Add their oil alternately with common oil. It is better to attenuate the mercury with saliva before using it here. When using it, rub in the ointment with salt. Leave it on for three days before bathing the patient. After the bath, anoint again. Repeat as necessary until cured.[32]

---

[32] The repetitious, curious and confusing phrases and the lack of order in these chapters reflect on the copyist of the Latin Ms. Dr. Stroppiana made a literal translation of it into Italian, whereas Tabanelli omitted many of these tedious sections. (LDR).

CHAPTER 43. BLACK MORPHEA

Our own experience and what we have learned from other sources confirm our statements that black morphea is incurable; we do not attempt it. However, we can try the recommended medicines used against serpigo, impetigo, itching, scabies etc.

Take two ounces each of tartar and soot; one ounce each yellow arsenic, alum and white and black hellebore. Grind them to a powder in a mortar. Then add handfuls of fumitory, wild clematis, herba flaura and wild mustard. Then take equal amounts of wild sorrel and ciclamen. Grind them to extract their juices. Then take three ounces each of soft palm and saracene soaps and mix them thoroughly with the powder. Then fold in the juices and the oil, a little of each at a time, alternately.

CHAPTER 44 EARACHE

The pain sometimes is caused by an influx of humors and sometimes to a worm or other foreign body. When the cause is pus, which is not hard like the pus of other abscesses[33] , we can deal with it. If you detect no foreign material (ie a worm, etc) and pain is the only symptom, use oil of musk placed in a scooped out half of an onion. Put the onion on some charcoal embers and let it boil. Drip the oil into the ear, as hot as can be endured by the patient.

Another prescription: Take rue and hard-boiled egg-white mashed together. The fluid obtained by straining it through a cloth is heated over embers and dripped in while hot.

Yet another: Take calamint, absinthe, cypress nuts and juniper twigs and boil them in water in a large bowl covered with a funnel. The steam is delivered to the ear of the patient who receives them inside a hood which covers his head and the funnel.

---

[33] Here the author suggests catarrhal otits with 'soft' pus (LDR).

If those measures fail you know that there is a worm or an abscess which is the cause. Additional signs are swelling, redness and local heat. Now you will need maturatives to bring on the pus as we described in the chapter on aposthems. Failing that you will know that the cause is a worm. We use the following to kill it and to extract it.

Take persicaria, both the leaves and the seeds, and grind them for the juice. Add some linseed oil and drip it in the ear. Use a forceps to extract the dead worm. You may use cupping to help remove the worm while still alive. But if the worm is securely ensconced, kill it by dripping in oil containing capers and calamint. If there are worms elsewhere in the body, mix white hellebore with wine and apply it on the part that hurts and it will kill the worm inside.

If a bean or a hair-ball [34] or other foreign body gets in the ear, apply a cup over the ear when the head is turned with that ear down-side. Provoke a sneeze to expel the matter by compressing the air toward the outside. Sometimes you may try to trap it with a twig or a wire, or you may introduce someting like terebinthe which will adhere to the foreign body and to the instrument that you insert and allow you to remove it. That method may frighten the patient and thereby increase his suffering. Therefore, I usually eschew it.

Addenda by Roland

A. Be reminded not to use cold remedies in the ear or hot ones in the eyes.
B. I recommend the combination of the cup and the vermicide.

HERE ENDS BOOK I

---

[34] I presume that this includes retained ear-wax (LDR).

BOOK II

THE NECK, THE NAPE, THE THROAT

Prologue

Let me not be accused of prolixity or of a vulgar style of writing simply because I seem to compress too much material in too few lines, leading to obfuscation and confusion, and causing difficulties in finding what one needs, so important for the user of a compendium. I will try to write not only for the well educated few but for the others as well. For them I plan to pass on all that the Great Doctor (ie Roger [35]) has taught me, in private as well as in public, and what I have saved in his notes. I will use a simple and a direct style of writing which will suit the larger group of readers, rather than one with a style better known for elegance.

After arranging and describing the full details of treatments for the maladies of the head, I will pass to surgical disorders of the neck and throat. I will examine in as great detail as possible the signs and the treatments of wounds, inflammations, scrofulas, glands, fistulas, goiters and, lastly, of internal ailments.[36]

---

[35] Hunt's Anglo-Norman Ms says 'my master' (LDR).

[36] These are the words of Guido II of Arezzo, the chief compiler and editor of The Chirurgia (LDR)

Chapter 1 Wounds Of The Neck

We treat wonds of the neck that were inflicted by swords or other sharp-edged weapons as follows. First examine them to find and to remove loose pieces of bone or other materials, using your fingers as well as your eyes. After clearing the wound suture it and dust on our red powder and follow with the topicals as described in Book I.[37]

When brisk hemorrhage or other complications prevent us from searching and removing as we intended, we close the wound (ie mass sutures for control), leaving gaps, awaiting an opportunity to clean out the wound through the openings. Then we complete the closure with sutures, except to leave an opening at the lower end. Then we proceed with the rest of our protocol.

When an arrow or another projectile penetrates through-and-through, from side-to-side, we insert a strip of bacon through the entire track. At the wound of entry we do nothing more for three days, or until good pus is discharged, than to promote suppuration using methods we have described, varying according to the season.

When good suppuration is in effect we replace the bacon with a cloth strip etc. as described (ie in Book I, Chapter 14). For all such wounds obey this precept: keep open the end until all the rest inside has healed. To that purpose, shorten the drain day-by-day as the interior heals.

---

[37] This method for primary suture of clean fresh wounds anticipated Hugh of Lucca (and Theodoric) in medieval surgical practice by more than a half-century. However, it was ancient, see Paul of Aegina (LDR).

Addenda by Roland

A. Some wounds are incurable. In that category are wounds that leak marrow from bones damaged by the weapon. However, damaged bone that does not leak marrow can be cured.

When using the fatty strips or other drains, do not insert them to the full depth where the drain can trap pus and cause it to enter the injured bone. Carefully lay in a larded cloth strip in the soft tissues up to but not beyond the edge of the wound in the bone. Then follow the prescribed routine.

Note this: The 'collo' (ie the nape) measures the 'nuca' (ie neck) to the level of the first spondyle (the spine of the first thoracic vertebra). The 'gola' (ie throat, the larynx and trachea) by definition enters the thorax, and lies between the two great veins in front of the nuca. The neck is defined in two ways. On one hand we describe the region on the sides between the head and the shoulders. On the other hand we describe the extent in front from the head to the interclavicular fossa (ie suprasternal notch). We use those terms to be precise in our descriptions of wounds and treatments.

B. When we remove the bacon we must insert two cloth drains, one from each end of the wound.

C. When both ends of the wound lie at the same level, suture only the middle of the wound and leave open both ends.

Chapter 2. Wounds At The Neck

When a wound by a sharp weapon cuts one of the organic veins [38], we do as follows. We pass a threaded needle under the vessel, avoiding the 'vein' itself, both above and below the site of injury and we control the bleeding.[39] Then we insert a moist (ie egg-white) cloth strip, without further enlarging the wound. During the winter months we continue the applications of a plaster until the purulent drainage

---

[38] These were the external jugulars

[39] These are ligatures-en-masse which included the perivenous tissues, and the overlying skin (LDR)

ceases. In the summer time we always use a dry strip covered with our brown ointment, etc. to favor the growth of healthy granulation tissue, just as we have treated other wounds.

When you see that the tissues between the cut ends of the ligated vessel are sloughing, cut them away (ie up to the ligatures) and apply topicals as above.

If a nerve has been cut crosswise or along its axis but has not been completely divided, you can treat it successfully if you do exactly as follows. Take some earthworms directly from the soil, alike in length and diameter to those we call lombrici. Chop them and boil them in oil. Apply the paste three, four or more times directly on the wounded nerve. A nerve that has been partially cut transversely may not heal even with this treatment. Yet, even without the treatment, the nerve will heal if you simply sew its covering membrane and apply the red powder. Therefore, treatment will not be useless. We can testify to cases where our treatments have succeeded, not simply to have the cut ends touching but by a secure union.

If the wounded region becomes swollen, return to the plasters you used at the onset and continue with them until the swelling subsides.

In wounds that do not injure the great vessels, you need only to insert a wet egg-white drain, and you do not have to shove it all the way in. Then (ie after the suppuration) you may continue with the other topicals.

Addenda by Roland.

A. If the wound enters an organic vein high in the neck, make two (ie mass) ligatures: one will be tied above the ear toward the front of the head. The other thread is tied distally, toward the shoulder and axilla. Similarly, if the wounded vein is at the mid-level or inferior or toward the midline, pass the ligatures under the chin and toward the axilla.[40]

---

[40] Roland's scheme for controlling the external jugular veins was to ligate the exposed vein under the mandible and lower down near the clavicle (LDR).

B. It seems that Roger believed that a transected nerve was beyond cure and he made no effort to bring together the ends and to sew them. However, we favor the following treatment which can provide a cure by the use of the cautery. Use a red-hot iron to touch the cut ends of the nerve and avoid contact with any other surface of the wound. Then use the paste of worms and, later, the consolidative powders and the rest, very much as we treat open fractures of bones. Furthermore, you should know that the cautery should be used in all wounds involving nerves and bones, as deep as they may be. For example, in a case of a projectile wound of the leg or of the shoulder, the cautery will stem the bleeding by shriveling the vein. And, an injured nerve, even when transected, should be cauterized before applying the topicals.

And know this: When nerves or large vessels (ie in the neck) are injured, you need not guarantee a full cure. Be satisfied to achieve free motion (ie of the head and neck).

C. Where Roger advises the use of egg-white I disagree. That is a naturally cold medicament. Nerves, arteries and veins are cool by nature and the use of cool medicines delays healing and lessens the chances for a perfect result.

CHAPTER 3. PROJECTILE WOUNDS IN THE NECK

When an arrow enters the neck and perforates an artery or vein and the hemorrhage is great, proceed at once to remove the arrowhead and close the injured vessel with sutures (ie ligatures or by mass closure of the wound) as described before. Then use our red powder. Or you may use a powder of dry donkey-feces. If dry feces are not available you may use fresh droppings which you have powdered by tossing them about in a cloth sac. This is how you make the powder. Take two ounces of frankincense, one of aloes, and sufficient amounts of egg-white and great mullein. Grind the dry stuff (ie including the powdered turds) and add some egg-white and mix in the mullein. Use enough in the wound to cause the arrowhead to come loose. The same effect is obtained with gypsum and grape seeds ground fine. Another good powder is made from ground flowers of daphne and charred ivory. Another: chew grains of wheat and apply them on the bleeding vessel, a useful remedy. Another, equally good: lime mixed with lye.

Once the bleeding is controlled, go ahead with the treatment.

Addenda by Roland

A. Note this: no matter where the wound may be, if a major vein has been cut do not remove your hemostatic medicines for three days.
B. Labdanum ground up with earthworms and mixed with egg-white is another good medicine for hemostasis, as well as for wound-care.
C. For contractures of nerves (ie tendons, sinews), use the milk of sheep and donkeys, always warm, to anoint the patient for nine days. If the site of the wound is where the patient can keep some of it directly (ie over the injury)—one thinks of a hand or a foot— the effects are even better. Then the applications can be made using butter or animal fat or mauve or oils of laurel and others, and warm ointments (ie the slippery materials will stay in place).

CHAPTER 4. WOUNDS OF THE THROAT

Those wounds are fatal which perforate or lacerate the esophagus or the tracheal artery (ie the trachea); even the wounds which injure but do not penetrate the organs. This holds for wounds by arrows and others. But, if only the outer membrane of the structures are pricked, the wounds are treatable as for any other wound.

Take care when you use hemostatic agents in treating injured veins not to remove the topicals until three days have passed.

CHAPTER 5. INFLAMMATIONS (APOSTHEMS)

Each of the different humors of the body may collect as super-fluidities in parts of the body, each with its own name. However, all the collections in common are called aposthems. There are four general types: phlegmonous, sanguinous and choleric of two sorts, one from normal reddish bile (ie choleric) and the other from abnormal black bile (ie melancholic). The latter gives rise to herpetic lesions (ie esthiomenes). Aposthems coming from phlegm are called zimia.

All aposthems have their own diagnostic signs. The sanguinous ones are red, the pulse is forceful and there are pain, heat and swelling. The phlegmonous ones are pale and soft and they are indented by the pressure of a finger. Red choleric aposthems are warm and reddish with a yellowish cast. Melancholic ones are very hard and tend to blackness in time.

Now we go to the treatments:

When an apostem is sanguinous, make a plaster of rue, cinnamon, lard, wheaten flour and onions. Simmer all for a long time in white wine and oil while continually stirring. Apply the plaster until the interior melts away and does not liquefy into pus. But if that does happen, carefully incise the mass at its lowest part. Use a knife and try to make the cut in the axis of the part (ie of the limb or torso). Use your fingers to press out the pus and then insert a cloth strip. Change it twice daily (ie until the interior has closed), and then treat the incision as you do other wounds.

CHAPTER 6. ANTHRAX AND CARBUNCLES.

When the lesion first appears apply cold compresses atop the lesion, using oil of roses and juices of henbane and grape tendrils, vinegar, worms and other cooling substances. Indeed, anthrax and carbuncles produce blood in excess (ie hot hyperemia). Apply well-ground scabious directly on the lesion—I recommend it.

I don't know how it works its miracles; it will destroy the anthrax and completely eradicate it. Bandage it on the lesion and leave it for an entire day. The cure is a complete one and no follow-up wound-care is required.

Addenda by Roland

A. The physicians (ie the clerics) recognize differences between anthrax and carbuncles which are of little concern for the surgeon. What we call the carbuncle is the hardening at the onset of the abscess, whereas the anthrax follows (ie when the contents suppurate).

I use treatments other than those of Roger. I use phlebotomy in the same region (ie during the carbuncle phase) to prevent metastasis (spread), while I apply rice-paste as the best topical. Before the induration increases I use cool topicals, as I do for quinsy. I avoid crust-forming astringents in noble regions or nearby, which will delay spontaneous drainage (ie the rupture of the abscess). Indeed, we must always get rid of pus in four categories of lesions: 1. When it is excessive. 2. When it is furious (ie necrotizing). 3. When it displaces (ie presses against) a noble organ. 4. When it impairs an important function.

In anthrax (ie after the carbuncular phase) as we do for other threatening aposthems, we apply cool topicals around the lesion and maturatives directly atop it. Remember, we should not use astringents on carbuncles and anthrax—here I refer to cases where the skin itself is fissured (ie about to burst). Only hot and dry topicals can work to bring the pus to a head and empty it. By acting like-on-like (ie a hot medicine on a hot lesion), its strength will overcome that of the threatening pus. The expulsion of the bad matter brought on by the continuous heat contributes much to the destruction of the anthrax. Therefore, continue by applying nut-shell paste on the pointing abscess.

Furthermore, much relief is obtained by drinking the juice of stinking iris.

I recommend the following plaster for both carbuncle and anthrax. Grind equal amounts of granular salt and dried figs and apply it for three days only on the blackening mound of the asbscess. When it splits open, lay on a poultice of wheaten flour, wild celery juice and honey until the slough is cleared away and there is no residual bad proud flesh. Then apply a powder of mastic and olibanum.

Chapter 7. Choleric Aposthems

Excessive accumulations of hot and heavy red bile causes chronic ulcerations after deep wounds. Our treatment is the same as that for anthrax.

Chapter 8. Aposthems Caused By Phlegmonous Bile

In such cases we resort to these plasters: Take eight ounces of malva roots cooked in eighteen ounces of hog-lard and two pints of spiced oil. Mince the roots and filter the oil. Then add nine ounces of fine flower of silver while stirring vigorously. Simmer over a low flame and make a plaster (ie to be applied warm).

Another plaster which also favors suppuration: Take malva, acanthus and early growth of althea (roots). Boil in water and grind with lard in a mortar. Then add butter, yeast, mothers' milk, tamarisk and a paste of flour. Apply it directly on the swelling to promote suppuration.

Another remedy: Take lily bulbs and heat them with lard and mash them. Reheat in an earthenware pot and add a roasted onion, yellow-horn poppy, ground cabbage leaves which have been cooked with lard, powdered linseeds which were cooked in wine and some other common maturative. If you apply the paste of the well mixed substances it will promote the maturation of a pus-filled abscess. When it is ripe, incise it where it points, just as we treat sanguinous abscesses.

Addenda by Roland

A. The plasters should be pastes (ie not poultices).
B. You can make a simpler plaster which may soften the aposthem and the nearby tissues as well as promote suppuration and relieve local pain. Take equal amounts of dry figs, lard and honey. Add the well boiled roots of althea to extract their essence and mix the fluid with the rest to make the plaster.

CHAPTER 9. CANCER[41]

The causes for cancer may be internal as well as external. The former include tainted humors; the latter include badly treated wounds. After four or five months an unhealed wound is called a fistula (ie hence a potential cancer). A cancer may be caused by something remote in time past as well as something recent. Furthermore, cancers involving nerve-bearing or vascular tissues must be treated differently from those in mostly fleshy locations. You cannot extirpate with a knife or a hot cautery a cancer in vascular and nervous tissues. Hippocrates said, "Those cancers should remain where they are. I advise against treating them; such attempts lead to a hastened demise." Be aware, then, that the neck, the nape and the throat are rich in nerves, veins and arteries which you must not cut or burn. However, you may treat them in other ways.,

For cancers of recent origin in those regions make a topical which is very effective, Take roots as follows: four ounces of bugloss, five ounces of sorrel, one ounce of celandine. Take one ounce of cinnamon, two of ginger, two of mercury and four of wine. Add sufficient amounts of pine resin and lard (ie to make a paste). Formulate the ingredients so: Mash the roots in a marble mortar and add the lard. Mix well. Grind the other ingredients together to make a powder (ie granules) and add the roots and lard. Heat the mercury and the resin

---

[41] Again I remind the reader that' cancer' is any chronic and necrotic ulcer, usually crusted over by a sloughing eschar. It involves the skin or mucous membranes and may be the result of ischemia, infection or neoplasm. Therefore, it is hard, dark and malodorous, and it may undermine the margins of healthier tissues. Only occasionally can we identify a true cancer by the medieval surgeon's description of invasion, permeation and vascularity of the periphery, as they give for cancers of the breast and testis (LDR).

in the earthenware vessel until they are melted, and add this and use it for an inunction.

If that is inadequate for curing cancers in vascular and nervous regions, apply this powder of white hellebore and aristolochium. After the cancer is arrested, lay on oakum pads wet with egg-white and green ointment. Finally, use the incarnatives which we will describe later.

Addenda by Roland

A. Temper the mercury with saliva or saliva plus ashes while you stir it briskly with a finger.

B. Apply crushed walnut shells on all cancers to suffocate them. Success will be indicated by the appearance of pure and thick blood and healthy granulations and when the cancer does not increase in size and thickness. However, a cancer that increases in thickness, even if the perimeter remains unchanged, has not been suffocated, and you must persist with your destructive medications.

C. You may use the following potion for good effect.[42] Take good amounts of pellitory, mustard-garlic, rue, thistle (roots), pimpernel, germander, agrimony, betony, elder (bark), clover-fern, fennel, asparagus roots, holly, hellebore (white and black), stinking iris, horse-radish, asclepia, dodder, marsh-reeds (roots), leeks (roots), carrots, ciclamen, pennywort (roots) and roots of fava-bean plants. The potion is equally effective against cancer, fistula, scrofula, bubo, glands, stasis ulcer (mal mortum), oily and scaly scabies, elephantiasis, podagra and chiragra (ie gout in the hands).

Boil all the roots and foliage in red wine until the volume is halved; then add a small amount of honey.

---

[42] This is one of the few prescriptions by a surgeon for a medicine to be taken by mouth. The amounts and the frequency of dosage are not stated. The complexity and variety of substances are not unusual for medications prescribed by the physicians, but such are seldom found in surgical treatises. (LDR).

Chapter 10. Scrofules Of The Neck

Scrofules appear in the neck, the axillas and the groins. The masses in those regions may be glandules instead of scrofules. To tell them apart grind clematis and leaves of citrons and mix them with oil, and let stand for three days. Apply it warm. Glands will regress. But if the area reddens and seems to need maturatives to bring on suppuration, use them. Then incise where they point.

If instead they harden and continue to enlarge during one to six months of observation, use this fresh oil: Take equal amounts of cleaned roots of thapsus and wild horse-radish and enough oil to equal the other two. Grind the roots and boil them in the oil. Introduce three or four drops into the ear on the affected side and allow it to penetrate. If the ear swells and then discharges pus that is a sign of success. Lacking that indication, persist with several doses of the oil and add this potion:[43] : use equal amounts of roots of marsh-reeds, ciclamen, bruscus, asparagus, white and black hellebore, peonies, valdemona betony, clematis, henbane, scrofularia, wild and domestic horse-radish and stinking iris. Take leaves of daphne and spirea and mash all the above together and boil them to reduce the volume by half. Have a young patient drink some once a day for a week, and dose an adult twice a day. Dilute every dose with an equal amount of wine, the total being one cup full.

If the patient cannot stomach the potion, add sugar and take care to warn him of the laxative effects. He can expect two or three passages after each dose. Sometimes you will make a point cauterization behind the middle cartilage of the ear. Do that during the time of a waning moon, eleven days before the new moon. During the same treatment he should take small servings (ie a small cake) of stinking iris or wild horse-radish every day until the moon has waned, alternating the the roots, one or the other each day. Of this treatment fails you must resort to the knife. No operations on scrofules or glands (ie in the neck) should be made by an inexperienced surgeon.

---

[43] The similarity with Roland's potion in the last chapter suggests that the copyist nodded in the repetition! (LDR).

Addenda by Roland

A. (After incising a gland) insert a cloth drain wet with egg-white. If any of the gland remains after three or four days, use the powder of hermodactyl or another corrosive. Treat the wound after the gland is gone.

B. If no swelling appears after the ear-drops the patient will not be cured.

Operations On Scrofules

To operate on scrofules and glands grasp the mass with your fingers and make your incision in the skin along the long axis. Peel back the skin from the mass with your fingernails to free the mass for extraction—not just the main gland but the others that are beneath it, not separating them; remove all as a single clump. On occasion bleeding will be heavy and you will have to delay while you pack the wound with soaked cloth strips.

If any of the scrofule remains, the next day apply the powder of asphodels just as we described in Book I in the chapter on scrofules of the head. Then get rid of the proud flesh and the pus.

In order to necrotize and corrode the tissues over the mass (ie when incision is not used) we apply the powder. When that wound is swollen and needs to be dried, fill it with egg-white-cloths with an oakum pad, also with egg-white, atop it all until the slough is macerated and the wound shows a little pus. Then we use the green ointment or others as described for treating the nose (ie polyps and granulation tissue).

Addenda by Roland

A. The transverse cartilage in the ear lobe is the one to cauterize specifically when treating scrofules.

B. The best plaster for eating away necrotic scrofules is this: Take roots of ferns and asphodel. Cook them in a good wine in which you have dissolved a small amount of sulfur. Make a plaster to corrode the scrofule.

Another good plaster for scrofules: Mince leeches in a pot and add lye and hog-bile and minced roots of bugloss . Mix well and apply after having the patient sip a raw egg in which you have mixed six or seven drops of euphorbia, if that is obtainable.

If none of the above succeed, go to a general purge and an opiate designed for the particular humor at fault. After the appropriate opiate has been concocted make a plaster of the roots of nettles and mustard boiled in vinegar. Add quicklime and lard and the plaster is ready (ie for scrofulas).

For glands, wherever they may be in the body and whether they be obvious or barely detectable, burn lead (ie litharge) with the wood of elder or fig or hazel and use oil and vinegar to make an ointment to rub over the glandule. Then bandage on a thin layer of cloth and a thin sheet of lead, and leave it for nine days. Remove it and renew the ointment. God willing, the patient will be cured.

If you consider the use of the knife in a region full of nerves , veins and arteries, such as the neck, the cut must be made with extreme care. Do not be hasty and do not act rashly lest you destroy the patient. Rather find a surgeon who will use the virtual cautery (ie corrosive topicals) rather than a novice or an unskilled operator.

Chapter 11. Fistulas

A fistula is an aposthem with a narrow orifce and a larger cavity at the other end. It may have internal or external causes. The internal causes include faulty humors, the external include unhealed wounds. The cause may be chronic or one of recent origin. The fistula may involve mainly fleshy regions or those containing many nerves, arteries and veins.

Each type of fistula has its own symptoms. Those in soft tissues drain watery pus while drainage from bones resembles washings from half-cooked meat. When the drainage comes from nerves it is dark.

Each type of fistula will require treatments suited for it and for where it is.

Here in the neck, nape and throat—regions rich in nerves, arteries and veins—we do not take risks with knives and cauteries. Instead, we do the following. We dilate the narrow external opening by inserting a strip of cloth covered with dry cyclamen, and we fill the entire tract, leaving it in place for an entire day or overnight. When the tract is dilated and there are not a lot of nerves and vessels, we introduce a rupturing medicine made from quicklime and lye. If the region has a lot of nerves we instead use a powder of asphodels. If the patient is very sensitive we use this special ointment: Take five ounces each of pepper, pyrethrum, yellow arsenic, mustard and an amount of palm soap to equal all the rest. Saturate a strip and insert it to the bottom of the fistula. This ointment melts away the scar from the opening down to the very bottom and destroys the fistula (ie the scarred lining) and dries it. When the watery pus becomes thick you will know that the fistulas such has been destroyed. Then do not delay in packing the defect with oakum wet with egg-yolk, or egg-white with oil until the inflammation subsides. Then use the green ointment for treating exuberant granulations. You may use other ointments to complete the treatments.

In places in the body which are not laced with nerves and vessels, even if the fistula is through-and through, insert a wooden strip as a guide to lift the overlying skin and cut it from the bottom toward the orifice with a bistouri and expose the full length of the guide. Then lay in a tent wet with egg-white and leave it a full day or overnight. Following that use the powder of asphodels. A brisk response with swelling is a sign that the fistula (ie the scarred lining) is gone. Then go on to treat the wound with egg-white and green ointment, etc.[44]

---

[44] The treatment with topicals was designed to corroded away the scarred lining and allow granulation tissue to fill the tract. In that fashion the surgeon converted a fistula, by definition a chronic wound, into a fresh wound, which he knew how to treat. If necessary and safe he laid bare the tract by incising along a guide. (LDR).

Addenda by Roland

A. Instead of ciclamen to enarge the orifice you may use roots of daphne, iris, briony, elder tree or wild watermelon.

B. A bubo is a mass in the axilla or groin which presents as a firm protuberance but has a profusion of roots going deep. It causes burning pain. Some of them are incurable. Indeed, when the patient suffers continuous burning in the region and he is very debilitated and the bubo is very large and when he feels pain deep in his chest—in cases of axillary buboes—that case is incurable. Furthermore, when those signs are observed and you can feel the soft centers and the overlying skin shows no sign of pointing, the case is not curable. However, when pus erupts and there is no retention of bad humors and the hard remaining mass has some soft spots and when you use corrosives (ie ill advisedly) and cause the mass to enlarge rather than to decrease in size, that case also becomes incurable. You should use maturatives followed by open drainage by wide incision. Do not delay the evacuation for any reason; a delay will compromise your chances for healing. Make your incision and use your medications as you would for abscesses and wounds.

CHAPTER 12. GOITER

Goiters grow in the neck. We treat them with this remedy. While singing the Pater Noster you uproot a young walnut tree (before it comes of fruiting age). Mash the roots with two hundred grains of pepper and boil them in a good wine until it is reduced by half its volume. Dose the patient every morning until he recovers. You may use other medicines: white briony, wild pumpkin, roots of cyclamen, oak fern, asparagus, bruscus, wild cucumber, cuckoopint arum and lungwort. Take marine sponge and acanthus (leaves) and butter. Obtain milk from a first-time whelped sow and roots of mullein. First let all the herbs dry before stripping and grinding them. Incinerate the sponge and the lungwort before grinding them and mixing with the others to make an electuary to place under the tongue at bed-time. Then boil some oak-fern in water with some cyclamen, betony and mullein until reduced to one-third of the original volume. At bedtime put some of the powder (used in the electuary) in this liquid and dose the patient. In the morning he should drink some of the fluid after it has been strained. And during the day of treatment the patient must abstain from drinking water. That abstention as well as not taking more of the potion or the electuary persists for three days. Then repeat the sublingual medication and etc. during the following six to eleven days.[45]

If those measures fail, you must proceed to surgery. If the goiter is a single nodule perforate it with a hot cautery (ie a wire) both in its long axis and across it and insert setons. [46] Then apply a cloth wet with egg-white and lard. Thereafter, twice a day tighten the setons until they cut through. Then apply our powder of asphodels to corrode the goiter. Then treat as you would other wounds.

If (ie after the overlying tissues have been cut by the setons) the goiter is not close to arteries, grasp it firmly with your fingers and carefully incise the capsule along the long axis and catch the nodule with a hook. Dissect away the surrounding tissues (ie shelling it out) to raise it to skin-level where you can use a finger to finish the extraction. Gently pack the defect with cloth strips, and control any hemorrhage as instructed in the chapter on arrow-wounds in the neck. Keep the patient at rest for three days. If any goitrous (the nodule) tissue remains in the neck use the corrosive powder of asphodels, followed with egg-white, etc. If you do not extirpate the entire goiter and a little bit remains tucked away, it will recur. Therefore, be sure of your clean-out before you suture the wound and use our red suture powder. Then follow our protocol for treating sutured wounds.

---

[45] Here is another example of an 'internal medical treatment for a surgical disorder (LDR).

[46] The wire cautery penetrates the tissues atop the nodule and the setons expose its surface, avoiding the risks of hemorrhage (LDR).

If the goiter is very large and the patient is quite old, do not operate. It will prove too difficult to dissect out, and we absolutely refuse to use a hot cautery in the region of pulsating arteries and of nerves. However, if some sort of operation must be attempted, be sure to securely tie the patient to a table to hold him, before you attempt any sort of intervention.

Addenda by Roland

A. Here is a valuable and effective medicine for goiter. Take four ounces each of peeled hemp seeds, sea sponge, lungwort, acanthus, tartar, bones of a bear (especially the skull) and squid's bone. Take two ounces each of peppers, ginger, rock salt, nutmeg nuts, cubebs, cloves, long pepper, white pepper, china-root, cinnamon, euphorbia, black and white hellebore. Also take samaras of elm, borax, cypress seeds, sea-shells and wild roses. Grind those to be ground (ie leaves and roots) and incinerate others (ie the bones and seeds, and make a powder of everything. Dose the patient in the morning on an empty stomach and at bedtime, taking as much as he can pick up with three fingers, and swallowing it bit-by-bit (ie as he licks it ?).Then make a plaster to place over the goiter, using powdered quicklime, brick-dust, dry figs and pumice. Boil the powders in wine and pour the (ie thickened) hot liquid on a hairy pelt and sprinkle powdered aloes on it before applying it hot.

I prescribe a diet of freshly baked leavened bread and small amounts of good wine, all to be taken for fifteen to twenty days. Repeat the medicines and the diet for another thirty days if you need it. I am confident of cures.

For young adults, ages fifteen to twenty, I fumigate the throat through a funnel and require an abstention from coitus for a year, and the refusal of cold meals and indigestible and fried foods and unleavened bread and plain water, all for a full year if possible, lest the goiter reappear.

After the fumigations, vigorously massage the goiter and the neck. If you treat royalty or wealthy patients massage with balsam. In lower-class patients use the yellow ointment. Lacking that you may use their own saliva or vinegar or warm wine.

You also may use this plaster: sorrel roots steeped in wine mixed with lard from hogs or, better, of bears. After blending and spreading it on a cloth sprinkle five ounces of ground aloes and apply it warm.

But the best results are obtained while the physician chants this prayer. "Flesh, flesh, flesh, go away, let the Son of God curse you. In the name of the Father, the Son and the Holy Spirit, go away from this person, your servant." Then he traces a circle around the patient's neck as he walks with a candle that has been blessed during the Feast of Candelora, while he sings the Paternoster three time in honor of the Holy Trinity.

B. You may use soapwort instead of mullein in the prescription.

CHAPTER 13 SQUINANCIA (QUINSY)

There are three types of quinsy which appear in the throat. First is the squinancia, although the word is also the general term for all three. This appears between the trachea and the esophagus and nearly always is fatal, excepting a Divine intervention. Second is called scinantia, when some of its pus is expelled to the outside, and it is less threatening. The third is quinancia. That aposthem is the least threatening because all the pus can be drained. The symptoms of all three include difficult respiration, both in and out, dysphagia for food and liquids, loss of voice and the inability to swallow saliva, which leads to constant spitting.[47]

Intervene as early as possible. When feasible, bleed the patient from a cephalic vein (ie in the arm) and a subungual vein, and have him gargle sapa or diamoron, or make a gargle of oak galls, pome-

---

[47] Squinantia probably was diphtheria; scinantia probably was a parapharyngeal abscess; quinantia probably was the true quinsy, a paratonsillar abscess (LDR).

granate, roses and lentils, all boiled in water. Use them frequently, because the gargles will cause the abscesses to point.

Meanwhile, as an external application, use dialthea or the like. You may make a plaster, best used for the second and third types, of elder-tree roots, leeks—not the foreign grown or the uprooted ones— absinthe, thistle and senecio. Mash them all and extract their juices. Take barley-flour and flaxseed powder and moisten them with enough of the juices to have a liquid which you can boil down to a thickness suitable for a plaster, which you apply hot over the painful area. Renew it, always hot, three or four times a day. When the abscess points inside the mouth, open it with a finger [48] or an instrument, and keep it open to drain the pus. An experienced hand will obtain a cure.

Addenda by Roland

A. Early in the course, persist with the repulsive gargle, and that usually will produce rheumatic (ie phlegmatic) humors. Then you can fall back on drying and astringent medicines to get rid of the humors. Use external applications of dialthea, etc.

B. Here is a plaster for type-three quinsy: Take malva and garlic leaves boiled in water, mash them with lard and make into a plaster. Or you may make one with bitter sorrel, garlic leaves and lard. Another, useful in such cases: Take half-cooked salted beef and chestnuts or hazel nuts. Tie a ball (ie a strip of beef wrapped around a nut) with a long cord to prevent it from being swallowed beyond recovery. After the patient swallows the ball the doctor jerks it out with enough force to rupture the abscess.

CHAPTER 14 THE TONSILS (BRANCHE)

The tonsils can swell within the throat and are like two almonds which make expectoration and breathing difficult. Early in the case

---

[48] An experienced surgeon often kept uncut one long index finger-nail! (LDR).

we rely on gargles. When they don't work we go to surgery. Sit facing the patient. Insert an instrument to hold open the mouth and depress the tongue so to expose the tonsil. Hook it with the proper iron or bronze instrument, and cut it with the special knife for that purpose, which leaves intact the capsule. Then have the patient use a gargle made of equal amounts of rose-water and vinegar, or you may use the juice pressed from planatins. If the bleeding is brisk, add mellicrate.

If there is pus, incise the capsule at the base and cut away the entire tonsil, roots and all.[49] Then you must control the bleeding with a gold or iron cautery.

Addendum by Roland

A. Another lesion appears near the epiglottis and is called foglio (ie leaf). It presents as one or more thin flat excrescences which obstruct the trachea and impede speech. When the patient opens his mouth to speak these flaps are elevated and cover the opening to the trachea, and when the mouth closes the laminae collapse and damp the volume and impair intelligible enunciation. That is when a surgeon's intervention is necessary.[50]

CHAPTER 15. THE UVULA

Not infrequently the uvula will swell or elongate. We treat that enlargement with astringent gargles and powders.[51] I use this powder: Take pomegranate flowers, oak-galls, peppers, pyrethrum and

---

[49] The first procedure simply scooped out some of the tonsil; the second was a more complete tonsillectomy. The instruments were designed specially for the procedure (LDR).

[50] It is clear that Roland had little knowledge of the nature and anatomy of the adenoids. His description of the obstructed airway suggests oropharyngeal tonsils. (LDR).

[51] A 'gargle" (Latin noun gargarisma) is an oral topical to sip and then retain or rinse about in the mouth. To "gargle" (Latin verb gargarizere) is to make the noisy irrigation of the throat, one way to use a "gargarisma" (LDR).

cinnamon and make a powder to apply with a narrow spoon-like instrument. I make the gargle with sweet wine or honey with similar amounts of vinegar in which I boil peppers, pyrethrum, larkspur and pomegranate flowers which I have ground. Have the patient sip some twice a day.

If that treatment fails, grasp the uvula with a forceps and cut it off at its thinnest port near the palate, carefully avoiding the base of the uvula itself. Warn the patient not to lie supine and to gargle with water in which someone has boiled a fat goose. I usually order the patient not to sleep (ie lying abed) for three nights after the procedure.

Sometimes before resorting to cutting I cauterize with a gold disc and use the gargles. You may also use a plaster made from equal amounts of warm honey, laurel berries, plums, pennyroyal, oregano and euphorbium. Make the plaster with oakum and place it on the dome of the head.

Addenda by Roland

A. Avoid reclining for sleep to prevent catarrh.
B. To reduce the swelling on the uvula I apply a (ie pointed) cautery to the occiput and a plaster made from heat-melted pitch containing powdered mastic and frankincense, applied warm over the occiput. Then I use an astringent gargle to block the accumulation of humors.[52] But if that should happen, I use gargles which are partly corrosive and partly detergive (solvents).[53]

CHAPTER 16. DISLOCATION OF THE CLAVICLE

If the clavicle is dislocated, deforming the base of the neck, and the end of the bone is thrust inward and down, and the surgeon does not intervene promptly, the victim may die of suffocation.

---

[52] Note the application of a defensive topical as a gargle within the mouth, to defend against the reaccumulation of edema - a phlegmatic humor (LDR).

[53] Roland does not specify them. I hesitate to guess what corrosives he dared to use (LDR).

With the patient supine have him open his mouth so you can insert a piece of wood between his teeth to maintain the gape. Then pull upward on his chin with a strap placed under his jaw, while you push downward on his shoulders with your feet. Continue the distraction until the sternoclavicular joint is restored. Then lay a plaster of malva or soldiers' ointment on sheepskin or oakum over the tender region. Reapply the plaster daily. Most often the reduction will be secure by the third day.

HERE ENDS BOOK II

BOOK III

THE TORSO FROM THE SHOULDERS TO THE GROINS AND UPPER EXTREMITIES

Prologue To Book III [54]

When I ventured to write a major work to be of use in these times, I wanted to pass on the teachings of our Master in the way he organized the topics—with an Introduction followed by a consistent arrangement of the contents. I have given much thought to making it useful for our contemporaries as well as for those who will succeed us, who will depend on my ability and my own good luck..

The prudent reader of this book should set aside his immediate interest (ie a case at hand) and not consider just his immediate needs. He will not give heed to picayune criticisms and he will attend to what has been written based on good common sense.

I believe I have arranged the work in large measure to allow one to find the various treatments separated into single sections. That will allow the avid surgeon more easily to commit them to memory.

In this Book III we will deal with treatments for disorders from the shoulders down, from the juncture of the neck with the thorax down to the genitals.

---

[54] Again, this is Guido of Arezzo's note (LDR)

Chapter 1. Wounds Of The Scapular Region

We treat a wound caused by a sharp weapon as follows: If fresh, we clean it and suture it, leaving an opening at one end. Then we dust on our red powder and follow with the treatments described in the chapter on suturing, in Book II.

If the wound is not recent, we first give it a good scrubbing to provoke bleeding (ie oozing) from the surfaces, and then we suture it.

In a wound caused by a penetrating projectile we introduce a strip of bacon and follow with the routine described in the chapter on projectiles.

Chapter 2. Wounds At The Sterno-Clavicular Joint

If a wound enters the joint, do this: Pack it lightly with a cloth strip or with oakum wet with egg-white. Follow that with a maturative plaster on a dry cloth to promote suppuration, varying it to suit the season (ie winter or summer).

Carefully remove any bits of bone etc. that you can find and use our black ointment. If the clavicle is fractured and if part of a bone or the joint itself is displaced, pull and lift the arm with one of your hands, and use the other to press the displaced bone into place. Then lay a pad over the reduced piece, wet with egg-white, atop which you place a bolster. Wrap it in place with a criss-cross bandage. Over that wrap a long bandage to elevate and hold the forearm (ie wrist) at the neck, taking care to take turns around a cushion under the arm at the axilla to keep the arm from slipping down. It must be kept in place until the recovery is complete.

If the wound is a compound fracture, leave an aperture in your wrappings through which you can replace drains and medications, to be used as in other wounds. An over-all bandage may cover the long bandage (ie with its opening).[55]

Chapter 3. Dislocation Of The Neck[56]

When the wound causes a displacement of the shoulder from beneath the cervical tissues, do this:

First clean the wound and scrape it to ooze blood if it is not fresh (ie when you first encounter it), and remove loose bits of matter; then suture it so: approximate the matching edges and take a deep bite (ie through-and-through) the lower edge and come out through the upper, and leave the needle in place. Then (ie to anchor the needle in place) wrap the protruding ends of the needle with the attached thread. Leave in the needle. Or, (ie instead of a single deep, suture-en-masse) you may use a row of needles taking smaller bites, each wrapped with its own thread, to obtain a neater closure. Then dust on the red powder and dress the wound, leaving open a gap at one end of the defect, as we do for other sutured wounds.

When we see that the edges of the wound are solidly joined, we remove the needles and threads. Progressively shorten the medicated drain in the wound, as in other cases. Remove the sutures and drains as you determine that the shoulder will not separate from the flap above it (ie not all at one time).

---

[55] This outer wrap is removed whenever the surgeon changes the dressings. The inner wrap, with its aperture is not disturbed. (LDR).

[56] The title is misleading. This is not a cervico-thoracic verterbral dislocation. Rather, it describes a 'saber-cut' wound which raises a flap over the shoulder and, as the flap retracts, it appears as if the shoulder is sliding away from the neck. The repair, using needles to transfix and hold the flap was not new with Roger. Some of the details in this translation are taken from H (LDR).

CHAPTER 4. LACERATIONS OF THE ARM, INVOLVING NERVES

When a wound transects a nerve or the bone in the arm, first lightly pack the wound with a tent soaked with egg-white, then replace it with a dry cloth and lay on a pack medicated according to the season. As usual, remove bits of loose bone, etc. Treat the nerve as we have instructed and apply the brown ointment and the others.

Addenda by Roland

A. If the bony fragments are not loose enough for easy and painless removal, leave them in place Make this paste which will loosen the bone or pieces of the arrow shaft: Grind polypodium with a little aged lard and bandage the plaster over the affected region. Or you may use the apostolicon because it contains attractive powders.

Another way to remove an arrow without pain: apply roots of saxifrage and marsh reeds with some honey ground to make a plaster. Be aware of the wound that oozes oily blood. That means that the marrow cavity (ie of the humerus) has been entered and that the wound will be fatal.

CHAPTER 5. SWELLINGS, TUMORS AND HARDNESS OF NERVES [57]

When nerves are painlessly swollen or are hard and contracted you have only to use a medicine of althea. Take two pounds of the gum of the roots of althea, one pound of greek-fennel seeds, five pounds of squills, three pounds of oil, one pound of wax. Take one ounce each of turpentine, galbanum, and gum of clematis. Take five pounds each of colophony and tar. Chop the roots and grind them; do the same with the linseeds (ie not mentioned in the foregoing),

---

[57] 'Nerves' included tendons, aponeuroses, ligaments as well as nerves (LDR).

fennel seeds and squills. Soak the mash in six pounds of water for three days. On the fourth boil the lot until the liquid is thick. Filter it through a cloth sack; you may add some hot water to facilitate the filtration of the viscous juice. Take two pounds of it with four pounds of oil and boil it until the water is gone. You will know that when the oil no longer floats. Now add the wax; when it melts add the turpentine, then the gum of the chopped clematis and galbanum, and, last of all, add the colophony and tar. Let it cool a while after taking it from the fire. It will be ready when a droplet placed on a marble tile spreads. Filter it again and save it. Rewarm it for use.

It is good for treating pleurisy and chest-pains due to cold. Rewarm about an egg-shell full, enough to anoint a healing chest. It warms the cold and moistens and softens the dry.

Chapter 6. To Clean A Suppurating Wound

If a foul wound begins to suppurate you may treat it with this ointment: Take one pound of oil, five pounds of ram's fat, two ounces of white wax , three ounces of greek tar, a large handful each of salvia, horse-mint, St.Mary's herb, soapwort, dill and rue. Mix the oil, lard and wax and strain them. Mix in the others which have been mashed and set it aside for use.

Another paste for the same purpose: Take a handful each of wild and domestic salvias, daphne, centinervia, saxifrage, artemisia and bugloss. Grind them in a mortar with one pound of ram's fat and make soft balls. Later on, drop a ball in a pound of oil and boil until the herbs precipitate. Remove from the fire and filter off the liquid. Boil it again before adding three ounces of wax in the summer, two ounces in the winter. When the wax melts add one ounce each of powdered mastic, olibanum, and colophony, while stirring assiduously with a spatula. Remove from the fire and stir in a little turpentine. Now you may set it aside for use. This ointment is very effective for cleaning away pus and for regenerating and nourishing healthy tissues.

CHAPTER 7. SUPERFLUOUS GRANULATION TISSUE IN WOUNDS

When proud flesh overgrows in a wound use a powder of hermodactyl dusted on a fluff of cotton soaked with saliva, which you stuff into the wound.

Another remedy: Take four ounces of quick-lime, one ounce of yellow arsenic and some warm water. Mix it well until everything is dissolved. Set it over a flame until it is completely dry. Grind the residue to make the powder, which you can save.

Another: Take equal amounts of hermodactyl, round clematis and verdigris. Grind them together to make a powder which will eat away the proud flesh without a violent action.

Another powder for use to corrode cancers: Take lime moistened with a little honey to make a paste which you shape into loaf and place on a tile. Grind it into a powder

CHAPTER 8. ERYSIPELAS IN A WOUND

Wounds may be complicated by several things, only one being erysipelas. The differential diagnosis and treatment for erysipelas follow here. Pustules may appear; the white ones are amenable to treatment, and they are a good sign. The black ones, usually hard, represent invasive erysipelas and carry an evil prognosis.

We should intervene with cool remedies. First lay on a pad wet with juices of house-leeks, henbane, stone-crop, umbellicus venus and hyoscyamus. Mix them with egg-white, oil of roses and white and red sandalwood oil. If you cannot obtain any of these ingredients, use what you have in the amounts available and do not go to something else. If the wound is excavated, fill it with the following: Take one pound of filtered lard, six ounces of colophony, four ounces of wax, two ampoules of oil and three ounces each of mastic, olibanum and myrrh. Mix the melted wax, lard and oil and filter them. Add the powders while grinding . When a paste is formed, use it.

Addendum by Roland

A. The excavation in the wound has three causes. 1. The original wound. 2. Failure to treat in the deeper region of the wound, thereby promoting the collection of pus. 3. The lack of skill on the part of the surgeon who treated only the upper part of the wound.

CHAPTER 9. CARBUNCLES FORMING IN WOUNDS

When you see a carbuncle forming in a wound, treat it repeatedly with the populeum ontment, made this way. Take one pound of poplar buds, five pounds of black peppers, three ounces each of belladonna leaves, the tendrils of blackberry bushes, hyoscyamus leaves, henbane, stonecrop, lettuce, leeks, sorrel, violets and cos lettuce and three pounds each of fresh hog lard (or well-washed older lard). Grind the poplar buds and mix them with the lard to make pills, and set them aside for two days. On the third day chop all the herbs and grind them well and mix in the pills. Leave the new pills untouched for eight days. Then break them in small pieces and warm them in a basin with a very fine aromatic wine until the liquid completely evaporates, all the while you stir it with your spatula. Spread the paste on a cloth and squeeze the paste to filter it through. Let it cool, and preserve it in a jar. This ointment works well against heat, acute fevers, insomnia (when applied to the temples) abnormal pulse (when applied to the palms of the hands and the soles of the feet. When mixed with the oils of violets and roses it will miraculously cool the part which is anointed. When rubbed in as a grease it will promote sweating.

An ointment specifically for carbuncles : Apply the following: Grind equal amounts of yellow arsenic and dry figs and mix with honey to the proper thickness. When you see the carbuncle recede and all that remains is the dead eschar, apply this ointment to make it come away. Take equal amounts of mauve, guimauve and acanthus, and mix them with lard, and allow to sit for three days. Then heat them and filter. Add some wax and mastic to the filtrate; filter again before using.

Addendum by Roland

A. Here I must emend Roger, whose method I do not approve. In these cases you should not use astringent substances

CHAPTER 10. INJURIES TO THE SOFT TISSUE IN THE ARM

When the flesh-wound is within three finger-breadths of either the shoulder joint or the elbow, the risks are great for complications and for an uncertain recovery. Wounds elsewhere in the arm are less serious.

In the regions near the joints black pustules may appear and the swelling may spread upward. But, if white pustules appear, the swelling tends to spread downward, and that is a good sign.[58]

The treatment here is the same as for other wounds that do not cut into or fracture bones

CHAPTER 11. WOUNDS OF BICEPS BRACHII [59]

If a tendon is cut along with its nerve and/or its muscle-belly, the case can be fatal. But, no matter if the wound transects the muscle or is in the long axis, press the wedges together and sew the wound.[60] Leave open a drainage space through which you may medicate and

---

[58] The juxta-articular deep wound may interrupt the arterial circulation and gangrene would ensue. But if the surgeon saw white pus and edema distal to the wound he sensed that the limb would survive, that is, the arterial circulation was sufficient to engender purulent inflammation and edema. The wounds here described were on the inner surface of the arm, where the vascular bundles were less protected by muscles. See the following chapter (LDR).

[59] Although the term 'lacertus' refers to the biceps muscle as a whole, here the reference is the lowermost part, the lacertus fibrosis over the antecubital fossa. A deep wound will divide the lacertus as well as the nerves and major blood vessels for the forearm (LDR).

[60] The closure here includes the skin and the panniculus, not the deeper tissues (LDR).

cleanse the wound. Follow that with our routine for treating sutured wounds. If erysipelas intervenes, treat it as above.

Be aware that a severe oblique contusion (ie not an open wound) which crushes muscular tissues in the arm can be fatal.[61] A vertical crushing blow can be treated with success.

CHAPTER 12. ARM-WOUNDS CAUSED BY PROJECTILES

When a projectile penetrates the arm through-and-through, insert a strip of bacon into both ends and treat them as we did for penetrating wounds in the neck. If the wound perforates only one surface, use only one strip of bacon etc.

Addendum by Roland

A. Take care to note if the projectile entered the bone marrow. In such a case omit the bacon, because an oily material is not to be used against the oily marrow. Furthermore, if the wound enters within three fingerbreadths above a knee or hand, the outcome will be fatal.

CHAPTER 13. WOUNDS WHICH CUT THE NERVES OR BONES OF THE HAND

When these wounds occur insert a single cloth strip as we use in wounds elsewhere in the body., Then, as in Chapter 11 above, treat meticulously. When necessary, tie the hand down on a table so to expose the interior of the wound. If only a nerve is cut [62], suture the tissues en masse (ie thus to approximate the ends of the nerve). Dust on our red powder. That method will allow the scar alone to miraculously reattach the cut ends.

---

[61] Imagine here a cudgel striking a crushing blow obliquely across the triceps and/or biceps (LDR).

[62] The term 'nerve' was applied as well to tendons. Both came to be called 'sinews' (LDR).

Addendum by Roland

The effect of cutting the nerves in the hand is the loss of the ability to open or close the fist. That may come from paying attention only to the superficial wound (ie the surgeon's failure).

CHAPTER 14. WOUNDS WHICH DO NOT CUT NERVES OR BONES

In such cases simply suture the wound and medicate it as described.

Not infrequently the accident is contusive (a serious fall) and there is a fracture. Then the swelling is conspicuous and bad humors accumulate (ie pus).You must eliminate it lest it harm the nerves, the flesh and the blood. Therefore, apply emollients to eliminate the pus and use gentle pressure (to squeeze it out), by flexing the forearm against the arm or the leg against the thigh. In other words, the goal is to get rid of all the pus before you proceed with medicating the wound.[63]

Addendum by Roland

A. In the cases of contusions (falls or blows), the first action should be phlebotomy. Then apply astringents (repercussives). If the initial effects are deemed inadequate, repeat the phlebotomies as often as necessary and reapply the astringents until the patient shows no further improvement. Then use diaphoretics and, if there is spasm, bleed him from two sites, above and below the injury.

If the swelling or mass persist at the elbow, you must incise and drain the pus after using maturatives. Incise where the topical brings the swelling to a point, near but not directly over the elbow. You want to avoid scarring (ie stricture) by draining the pus from a nearby site.

---

[63] Here, again, the surgeon eschews the knife and does not incise to drain the pus. He applies corrosives (emollients) to eat through the skin and uncover the abscess. Having created a wound, he then sets about to treat it (LDR).

Chapter 15. Dislocation Of The Humerus At The Shoulder

We intervene as follows. Place the patient supine and use a pear-shaped object, wood or stone, wrapped with a lot of yarn. Place it in the axilla and put your unshod foot on it. While pulling the arm guide the humerus into its proper place. Before releasing the arm, cover the entire area with a cloth wet with egg-white and secure it with a long bandage. Then release the traction on the arm. Put a cushion under the arm and bandage it to hold it in the reduced position.

If the reduction does not hold after three days, reset it, anoint it and rebind it. If humors are superfluous (ie edema), bleed from the opposite arm.

If this method fails, take a long and rather wide board and cut a notch to accept the wrapped ball and the arm over it at its widest part (ie the axillary folds) while two assistants hold the board upright. The patient is seated or stands on a stool to which is tied a strap. While the surgeon pulls down on the arm, another assistant jerks away the stool from under the patient, who now is suspended and the dislocation is reduced. Now bandage the arm as above.

When the patient is a child, place a pad in the axilla and push on it with one hand while you pull up on the arm with the other. That will restore the joint. Then apply a fomentation of water containing viscous mauve, dialthea and soldier's ointment. Cover that with an oakum pad, held in place with bandages.

When the reduction is perfect (ie in adults), immediately apply this astringent: Mix our red powder with egg-white. Add wheaten flour and dip a wooden paddle in it, and smear on enough to cover the region; then apply a wrapping. Leave it on until the reduction is secure. If the bandage is too tight and edema is apparent, put the patient in a warm bath and remove the bindings. Sluice him with the warm bath while he is in the tub. When he is better, apply this plaster. Take powdered mastic, olibanum, greek tar, bol'darmenie, wax and ram's fat. Melt all, soak a cloth in it and lay it on warm. You also may use the apostolicon.

Addendum by Roland

A. Be sure that the humerus (ie the head) is not fractured before you undertake to reduce a dislocation. You must not separate the two fragments and allow an influx of humors into the joint.

CHAPTER 16. DISLOCATIONS AT THE ELBOW

When the elbow bones are separated at their normal joint, do this. Lay a strap across the bend of the elbow and continue it around your foot as a stirrup. Then flex the forearm toward the arm while you manipulate the bones into place. Flex and extend three or four times until you are successful. Then suspend the forearm from the neck, holding it flexed to prevent a redislocation.

After a few days, let the patient try to flex and extend the forearm, but continue to use the sling, allowing some freedom of motion.

Addendum by Roland

A. Another method: Extend the forearm on a flat horizontal board. The surgeon sets his heel over the elbow while he manipulates the bones into place. Then attach a small splint, and take care not to impair the nourishment of the limb.

CHAPTER 17. DISLOCATIONS AT THE HAND

In such cases, the surgeon grasps the forearm with one hand and the patient's hand with his other. Gently and firmly he replaces the bones into their proper positions. He may use fomentations and inunctions to help. Then he binds on a small flat splint. The same method is used when there are wounds with dislocations.

CHAPTER 18. FRACTURES OF THE ARM AND FOREARM

When a forearm bone or humerus is fractured exposing the marrow cavity the injury is life-threatening.[64] When the marrow is not exposed a cure is possible.

In the first place, do not fear the injury to the soft tissues. Simply realign the bones by grasping on both sides of the fracture and distracting them gently and carefully by pressing them in place if at the wrist. If the fracture is in the forearm, use an assistant to pull on the fingers against traction on the forearm. He may also pull on one end of a humeral fracture while the surgeon manipulates the fragments. Then use a four-finger-breadth wide bandage to hold them in place, over which apply an egg-white-wet cloth covering the whole region. Then wrap another bandage, over which you arrange splints to suit the case. Hold them with cords for three days. Then repeat the dressing three times. On the ninth day apply astringents, such as our red powder; it serves as well as an inunction. Then replace the splints and bindings. The limb should be continuously protected against displacement for several days, until the bones are securely united (ie by callus).

Be sure that the dressings are not too tight and cause swelling. In that event, put the patient in a warm tub-bath and foment him with warm water containing mauve, acanthus, etc. Then rub him dry.

If the union is good, anoint the site with dialthea or soldier's ointment, and apply oakum pads held with bandages and cords.

If the union is questioned, reapply the astringent powders and observe. Once united, repeat the daily inunctions, fomentations and bindings until the cure is complete.

If inflammation (ie erysipelas) is apparent beneath the dressings, remove them and treat that as previously described.

---

[64] A wound which cuts deeply enough to enter the shaft of a long bone will have divided all the soft tissues, including the major vessels and nerves. The surgeons recognized the awful consequences of a gangrenous limb, and they saw the leakage of bone-marrow as the evil omen (LDR).

CHAPTER 19. COMPOUND FRACTURES

In that case you must use assistants to support both ends of the limb while you explore the wound with a finger. Immediately remove all loose fragments and realine the long bone. Apply splints, as described above, and use the egg-white-wet wrapping, leaving an opening in it as well as in the overlays.

The straps (ie which bind the splints) should include the entire region except where they pass over the wound. Leave a gap into which you place a wet cloth drain. Change it daily and follow our routine of wound medications. Loosen the bindings every three days until the wound heals. Then you may use fomentations, etc.

CHAPTER 20. MALNUTRITION

You may encounter aged or debilitated patients who cannot generate enough nutritive power to heal their injuries, leading to malunion (ie by callus) of the fracture and the attendant pain and suffering. Use this plaster in such a case: Take equal amounts of greek tar, naval tar and resin, all melted together and applied as hot as is tolerated. Bandage it with a light hand.

CHAPTER 21. MALUNION OF FRACTURES

If after three or four months the patient returns to the surgeon with a malunion, begin by using the fomentations, and repeated them three or four times. When he shows some improvement (ie less local pain), refracture and re-set the bones and treat as before.

Chapter 22. Cancers, Fistulas And Other Aposthems Which Appear

We will not repeat much of what already we have said about these subjects. Treat open wounds with the cited ointments. In nerve-rich regions of the arm you may use the powder of asphodels as well as the ointments. Be sure to distinguish a fistula [65] from a cancer. It is better not to treat a cancer in that case, In regions that are not rich in nerves or tendons you may treat a cancer by cutting it away and cauterizing the margins of living tissues with a hot iron. Then use a mixture of egg-yolk and oil until the inflammation caused by the cautery the subsides. Then go to the green ointment, etc.

Addendum by Roland

A. Another treatment for cancer: Take finely ground myrrh and aloes. Grind out the juices of plantain, absinthe and celandine in a mortar and mix with the powders before applying.

Fistulas In The Arm

In fleshy regions go to the ointments, incision and cautery and follow with medications.

Bone Corroded By A Fistula

Here you must get rid of the rotten bone. Remove it (ie scrape it away). Then treat as described above and elsewhere.

---

[65] The term fistula included chronic ulcers which drained foul stuff, not needing an internal source other than the infected material within the ulcer. The categories of necrotic, crusted, chronic sores were labeled cancers (ie also as gangrene), fistulas and ulcers. The latter simply were wounds which did not heal for thirty or forty days (LDR).

CHAPTER 23. WOUNDS OF THE THORAX.

Transverse wounds caused by swords or other cutting weapons should be closed by sutures. Then use our medications.

If the wound penetrates, insert a wet cloth drain and proceed as in other wounds. If blood or pus enters the chest, secure the patient to a plank so you can twist and turn him to favor the escape of the stuff out the wound. Keep it open until the cure is complete.

You need not suture vertical wounds. Dressings with medications will be sufficient.

Addendum by Roland

A. Here is how I bind up a chest wound. Perforate one end of the bandage and slip one arm through it. Carry the wrap under the opposite axilla and around the entire chest and over but not under the arms. Tie it . Or you can split the bandage and tie it over the unbound arm.

However, I prefer the perforated bandage to the split-end method, because it is more adjustable (ie easy to tighten or loosen). But, use your own judgment and follow your own authorities.

CHAPTER 24. WOUNDS CAUSED BY METAL WEAPONS PENETRATING THE CHEST OR BREAST

When the wound is round (ie not a flanged or barbed arrow) remove the weapon with a light hand. If the wound is subcostal or intercostal you may incise between the ribs and insert a wedge to facilitate the extraction. If that doesn't work, it will be better to leave it alone. If the penetration is partial (ie not through-and through), the insert a strip of bacon and follow with the medications used elsewhere. Do not forget to insert a tampon made in a way to facilitate grasping and removing it without risk of further injury (ie rolled and bound with a dangling thread).

Addenda By Roland

A. It is better to use a tampon even if there is no fear that pus will collect that after removing the bacon strip.
B. Use a long many-tailed bandage if the operation involves the abdomen as well as the thorax. Leave the ends of the bandage outside and easy to find.

Chapter 25 Greenstick Fracture Of A Rib

When the fractured rib is bent inwards, place the patient in a warm bath and spread honey over the fracture, using dry hands. Or you may use turpentine or viscous malva. Press down on the fracture itself and release it suddenly. Repeat the action until the rib has straightened. You may apply a cup to achieve the same result.

Then apply apostolicon or a similar plaster.

If there is an open wound anywhere over the belly or groins and the intestines are not eviscerated or damaged, treat that wound as you do for one in the chest, whether or not a weapon head had penetrated (ie the abdominal wall); whether or not the entry wound is a round puncture or if it is a linear incision, vertical or other.

Chapter 26. Wounds of the Heart, Lungs, Stomach and Liver.

Wounds of those organs and of the diaphragm are beyond our abilities. When the heart is injured, the lethal signs are: hemorrhage of foamy blood and gasping respiration; deep and gasping breathing when the diaphragm is injured; wounds of the liver reflect its damaged functions and the liver itself is directly observed; a wounded stomach spills its contents. As I say, all these wounds are mortal. Therefore, to avoid accusations that your interventions caused the death, decline to undertake treatment.

CHAPTER 27. WOUNDED SPLEENS

The spleen is an accessory organ; you should not willingly undertake to treat it with the knife. If it is wounded, treat it with our usual routine of topical applications.

CHAPTER 28. HERNIATED LUNG THROUGH A WOUND

When some lung protrudes through a slit-like wound you may fear that you will do more harm by enlarging the incision. Our method (ie to the contrary) consists of placing the patient flat on his back, completely extended. Grasp the upper wound-edge while an assistant takes the lower edge. Both of you simultaneously pull up on the body while the patient holds his breath. Of a sudden, the lung will pop back in.

CHAPTER 29. INTESTINE EVISCERATED THROUGH A WOUND

When the eviscerated lacerated gut is otherwise quite healthy, no matter the angle of its wound, do this. To prevent cooling of the extruded viscera before you can begin your operation, split open the belly of a living animal and lay its warm viscera over the patient's wound. That will help in its recovery.

Then take a tube of elder-tree bark with about the same diameter as the wounded loop, and about an inch longer than the wound in both directions. Completely insert the shaved-thin tube through the opening into the lumen of the intestine and close the wound with sutures. That will allow unobstructed passage of the intestinal contents and will not interfere with the healing.

Then repeatedly irrigate the soiled intestine with warm water squeezed from a sponge. When it is nicely clean, return it into the belly, by fully extending the supine patient and gently shaking him (ie bound to a plank during the operation).[66] You may have to en-

---

[66] Bruno and other medieval authors advised flexing the patient while he is immersed in a warm tub, and shaking him (LDR).

large the wound to relieve an incarceration. Once in, inspect it for damage through the open wound. Then sprinkle in the red powder once a day. When you observe clean healing inside, close the outer wound with sutures and use our topicals.

When the wound is very large, we add a large tampon in the treatments. We lay it full-length in the wound with both ends protruding. We close the outer layers loosely over the tampon and use our powders, etc.

Every day we pull out a little of the tampon from the lower end and we renew the wet cloth compresses. When we see that the skin wound has sealed over it we remove the tampon and continue with the medications, taking advantage of the persisting opening after the removal.

During the time of the treatment we prescribe an easily digestible light diet.

CHAPTER 30. FISTULAS, CANCERS AND OTHER APOSTHEMS

We will repeat what we have stated before: When these lesions appear in fleshy tissues we cut, we burn and we apply ointments and powders.

But we add this proviso: When a fistula communicates within the abdomen (ie fecal, etc.) do not use the powders and ointments which will offend the innards. Simple dilate the fistula (to favor free drainage) with strips of cyclamen. Lay the patient so positioned on a pallet that the fistula will drain freely. Then insert drains wet with corrosives and other medications to follow.

CHAPTER 31. CANCERS OF THE BREAST

The following deals with the specifics of cancer of the breast. When the breast is hard and dark and burns painfully, it is beyond cure by extirpation. If only a part of the breast is involved you may be able to treat it first with a corrosive powder of asphodels and emollients (ie corrosives), and you may try to excise it.[67]

---

[67] Rather than cut into the breast to expose the mass, the chary surgeon "ate his way" through the skin and panniculus with corrosives. Or, if the cancer had eroded and ulcerated, the corrosives would act on it. Rare successful ablations have been reported (LDR).

Addendum by Roland

A. Use this corrosive powder, as an escharotic, to destroy cancers and fistulas. Take yellow arsenic, verdegris, elder tree sap, rock salt, and the incinerated following: deer-horn, hare-bones, human feces, sangdragon , river-crabs and powdered leather. And take tartar, salvia, quick-lime, dried penny-wort, black pepper, aloes, ginger, frankincense, mastic, nitrum and alum. Make a powder.
B. First wash the region with a baby's urine or vinegar or water in which you have soaked the bark of an acorn-oak. Then liberally dust on the powder.

CHAPTER 32. INFLAMMATIONS OF THE BREAST

Breast abscesses appear when menstruation is blocked. Normally, the spongy mammary tissues soak it up and turn it to milk. If the milk does not flow it remains trapped and makes the breast tissue hard and excruciatingly painful.[68]

Do this: Apply emollients (ie non-corrosive) such as malva, acanthus and the like. When the abscess points, incise it and insert a long-tailed drain until the pus is all gone and you can cleanse the defect. I insist on a long-tailed drain because more than once I have seen a drain sucked into the abscess where it becomes the source of suffering and requires an incision to find and remove it.

CHAPTER 33. INVERTED NIPPLES

We see this in primiparas and in other recently delivered mothers. They cannot nurse their babies, who then waste away. You have to apply cups over the nipples to evert them and allow the babies to suckle. Use followup treatments known to you.

---

[68] A simple explanation why amenorrhea and lactation occur together after parturition (LDR)

CHAPTER 34. WOUNDS OF THE PENIS

These wounds are to be sutured as any others. The same holds for the scrotum. If a testicle extrudes, replace it, close the opening with sutures and apply the red powder, etc.

Addendum by Roland

A. A transverse cut which does not enter the urethra can be repaired by suturing the separated parts of the penis end-to-end. However, a suture-repair of the urethra may not succeed because the acidity of the urine may reopen the wound.

Cancer Of The Penis

If there is no proximal invasion, you may amputate the entire diseased part, including some normal tissues beyond. Then apply a hot cautery, iron or gold, and follow with the medications.

CHAPTER 35. FISTULAS OF THE PENIS

Treat here as for fistulas elsewhere: emollients [69] (ie corrosive),etc. If a crusted pustule appears (ie blocking the drainage) use the white ointment in which you substitute rose-water and violet-oil for the vinegar and common oil.

If the penis itself is ulcerated with erosion of the cord (ie fibrous septum), causing edema and swelling and induration, apply oil of violets with egg-white on the surface as well as inside. If the external meatus of the fistula is too small, insert a strip of wax, or other, to favor drainage of the pus.

Another remedy: Aloes, wild celery juice, oil of violets and egg white, mixed and applied.

---

[69] Another reminder that an emollient used in a fistula was a corrosive. It 'softened' the dense scar which lined the chronic fistula by eating it away (LDR).

CHAPTER 36. ULCERATION AND SWELLING OF THE SCROTUM

When redness and swelling occur, take iron filings, juniper-tree sap, myrrh, colophony, betony and resin. Grind finely and mix with hot oil, adding the resin and the amalgam together. Wash the scrotum with hot water and apply the ointment on the inflamed area.

Another effective remedy : hulled beans, as cooked for eating.

Another: Minced stone-crop and dill, with oil of violets, then add egg-white. Or use egg-white and violet-oil alone.

Addendum by Roland

A. Sometimes warts and crusts grow on the penis. Destroy the warts with powders of asphodel or hermodactyl. After removing the warts, treat the crusted defects as wounds. First foment with viscous water of malva, acanthus, etc.

CHAPTER 37. RUPTURE OF THE SAC[70]

The sac is the membranous tissue which encloses the viscera and prevents them from escaping through the openings which remain after the hernia is reduced, varying in size from a small nut to a large egg-shaped bulge. The opening may allow intestine to slip down along the spermatic cord as far as the testicle.

When this rupture is recent and is reduced, and the patient is yet a young boy, make a truss which presses on the opening, and administer eleven little loaves of comfrey and egg-yolk, to be eaten during eleven days preceding a new moon and into it, one a day.[71]

When the hernia is large (ie an indirect hernia), no matter the age, the treatment includes cutting and cauterization.

---

[70] This is the simple hernia ventosa. The hernia is a local bulge, presenting as a gas-filled knuckle of bowel (LDR)

[71] Another rare example of an internal surgical medication (LDR)

Set the patient on a tilted bench, head and shoulders down, legs and thighs up, to favor drift of the intestines toward the chest. Carefully displace the scrotal contents toward the hernial opening and mark its circumference with ink or charcoal. Grasp the entire skin, cord and contents (ie the sac contains no viscera) and burn through the mark in the skin all around. Then insert the cautery through the cord and membranes from side-to-side and from front to back and insert thin wooden strips as you withdraw the cautery. The strips will transfix the cord. Place a tough thin cord under the crossed sticks and tie it down as tightly you can. Then, with great care, using three applications of the cautery (ie for continuous intense heat) burn through, just beyond the sticks.

The rupture may be empty (ie a direct hernia). In that case you may include the membranes over cord, tracing the ink-mark with your cauteries, side to side, up and down, stripping the membranes, and always triply burning.

Then, incise the membranes over the opening lengthwise and strip away the underlying cord and membranes which you divide with your cautery. Lay an oakum pad with egg-white over the opening and move the patient to bed with his legs continuously elevated, binding the legs and the thighs together to prevent them from spreading apart before the local inflammation subsides.

Use the red powder and astringents, then the apostolicon. Maintain a light and digestible diet.

After the wound has healed, use a truss for two or three months.[72]

CHAPTER 38 SCROTAL HERNIAS

When the intestine falls into the sac, first of all replace them into the belly. If that is a difficult task, administer a clyster or purges and

---

[72] As I interpret the text, the surgeon ligates the spermatic cord and its membranes and the sac but does not remove the testis. In the following chapter, when dealing with a scrotal hernia, he does remove the testis with the sac. However, Tabanelli sought explanations in the commentaries of Roland and in the Glosses of the Four Masters (T. p.85 ff.). He suggests that Roger et al. really dissected the hernial sac and membranes, ie cremasteric, etc., and isolated the spermatic cord rather than ligating it. Roger's text alone does not agree with that hypothesis (LDR)

massage over the sac with emolliemts. After replacement, operate as for the hernia above, with an assistant plugging the hole with a finger to keep the intestines inside while you make your incision around the membranes to bring out the testicle and strip the cord.

If you encounter gas in the cord, return the herniated loop into the abdomen before tying off the cord twice. Lay the ligated testicle on a small board and cut it off between the ties and cauterize the ligated stump strongly, three times.

Then dress with an oakum and egg-white pad. Keep the patient in bed for nine days, with daily dressings of egg and oil. The inflammation will subside and the cord will come away. Then the patient can foment himself with boiled acanthus, pellitory, absinthe, etc. Then use the other topicals.

CHAPTER 39. HERNIA[73]

Hernias form from the humors which descend from the kidneys to the testicles. You can tell what it is by palpation.

Here you incise the ,membranes over the testicle and release the water. Then you insert a drain and wash out the defect.

However, if you wish to avoid a recurring problem first ascertain if the fluid is or is not purulent. If it is watery, leave it alone (ie do not incise). If it is purulent, do as above, and treat your incision as any wound.

CHAPTER 40. FLESHY HERNIAS [74]

These are abnormal fleshy accumulations near the testicles. They involve the adjacent membranes. As soon as it is detected, excise it with a cautery along with the cord (ie through a scrotal incision) up to the ring. Then close the opening with sutures and follow with our usual medicaments.

---

[73] This is hydrocoele (LDR).

[74] These are neoplasms of the testes or epididymes, the so-called herniae carnosae (LDR)

Addendum by Roland

A. Occasionally the carnosity invades a loop of intestine (ie a ventosity). In that case reduce the distension with medicines: the juice of St. John's wort is an effective potion.

CHAPTER 41. STONE IN THE BLADDER-NECK

Make the diagnosis as follows. A seated sturdy assistant holds the patient on his lap, A strap binds the patient's ankles and passes under the assistant's arms and behind the patient's neck.(ie the knees and the thighs are flexed and the thighs are abducted). The surgeon, seated facing the patient, inserts two fingers of his right hand into his rectum and presses down hard on the suprapubic region with his left hand. Between the push of the hand into the bladder and the lift from below he can feel the stone as a dense and weighty mass, not as a soft fleshy urinary obstruction (ie the prostate).

Addendum by Roland

A. When you suspect a stone, administer diuretics and stone-solvents. If those fail to relieve the symptoms, you can be sure that a stone is not the cause.

CHAPTER 42. DISPLACING A STONE FROM THE BLADDER-NECK

When you seek to relieve the obstruction at the bladder-neck by displacing a stone, first use fomentations and inunctions, and insert some oil via a syringe. After a brief wait, insert the syringe all the way to the bladder-neck. Then, very gently and carefully push the stone back into the bladder.

Ours is the most reliable and the least distressing technique. First we foment and anoint. Then we examine (ie as above) and make certain the diagnosis with the bimanual method, and we gently displace the impacted stone, carefully pushing it down and back. You will provide lasting relief.

CHAPTER 43. SPECIAL PRECAUTIONS FOR REMOVING BLADDER-STONES

Always limit the diet in preparation, and have the patient eat almost nothing for two days before the operation. On the third day , having established the diagnosis as we described, you push and hold the stone in the bladder neck with the intrarectal fingers while you cut down on it through a vertical incision in the perineum, and you extract it.

Dress the wound for nine days with twice-daily fomentations of acanthus, pellitory and malva, and use topicals of egg-yolk on oakum pads in the winter. In the summer use whole eggs.

Addenda by Roland

A. Do not enforce the dietary restrictions if the patient cannot fast or is feeble or is a child.
B. Take care not to cut the central perineal ligament. Always incise on one side or other.

CHAPTER 44 SUPERFLUOUS PROUD FLESH AT THE BLADDER-NECK INCISION

The accumulation (ie after lithotomy) is removed with a sharp knife, and the defect is closed with sutures. Then medicate.

Take special care: If the stone is so large that you cannot extract it, treat it only by displacing it, as we have instructed.

CHAPTER 45. WOUNDS OF THE BACK WHICH INVOLVE THE SPINAL CORD AND NERVES

We will not repeat the material dealing with the dorsal regions (including the bladder) except to mention that vertical wounds deep into the back which may involve a nerve can be treated. But you treat in vain a wound which transects the spinal cord.

CHAPTER 46. WOUNDS OF THE RECTUM

When a sword or other sharp weapon cuts into the rectum in its long axis, treat it as an ordinary laceration. But if there is a transection with complete or partial retraction of the cut ends, tie off the open end of the rectum with a sturdy cord to block the feces. Keep the sturdy ligature in place until the tissues beyond it slough away. Then treat that wound with our medications.[75]

When the rectal wound does not penetrate, an ill-advised medication (ie probably a corrosive) will make matters worse.

If the weapon is a projectile, treat the wound as a laceration.

Addendum by Roland

A. The longano is the end section of the rectum, between the sacrum and the coccyx, including the ampulla (LDR).

CHAPTER 47. WOUNDS OF THE KIDNEY

These are rarely encountered. Such cases are best trusted to divine interventions rather than to the surgeon. However, if he is conscientious he may be able to be of some help, taxing his ingenuity according to the magnitude of the injury. If a fistula ensues, he may treat it in the ways he now knows.

---

[75] The consequences of this treatment are beyond fantasy (LDR).

CHAPTER 48. PERIANAL ABSCESS, CARBUNCLE, CANCER AND FISTULA

An abscess may appear near the anus and present itself as a hard ball, a carbuncle, which may drain spontaneously and then re-form and become a fistula. In your initial assessment ask the patient if flatus escapes via the fistula; that will indicate an opening within the rectum. Treat it so:

Insert your greased long finger and explore within the rectum especially to feel if a probe can easily be passed from outside through the inner opening of the fistula.

If so, thread a seton, using the probe as the needle, and tie it in place. On a later day cut down on the probe. If you wish to avoid cutting, introduce a good amount of corrosive ointment along the tract, as you tighten up on the seton. When it is laid bare, treat the defect as an open wound.

CHAPTER 49. HEMORRHOIDS

There are three types: 1. The Internal, causing bleeding and pain. 2. External, with or without pus. 3. Enlarging clusters, resembling figs, which are very constrictive (ie sphincter-spasm) and painful.

When hemorrhoids are internal, you should make them empty their blood, first fumigating the region to relieve the pain. Use mullein, marrubium and horsemint, and take chestnut shells, pumpkin rind and old shoe-leather. Set all on hot coals to create fumes over which you seat the patient on a perforated bench. Repeat the treatments until the bleeding stops and the pain subsides. Then apply leeches to complete the treatment.

In treating the external clusters use an instrument as for a clyster. Inject the juice of wild watermelon to be retained for one or two hours. Repeat until the burning discomfort subsides. Then anoint with white ointment made without vinegar. Then fumigate as above.

When external hemorrhoids enlarge and no pus appears, take

the leaves of artemisia and absinthe and grind them and boil them in linseed oil. Apply that as hot as the patient will accept, for three or four days. This usually is a good remedy. But if you do not observe any shrinkage, place some honeysuckle fruit in an earthenware pot and incinerate it and make a powder of the ashes. Apply it after you anoint the piles with honey. Then rub on raw sheep's wool with your hands (or feet!). Apply the powder immediately. Continue the measures until the hemorrhoids no longer shrink.

If later on you want a complete cure, ligate each 'grape' with a silk thread. When the region is not sensitive you may cut off the pile. If not numb, let the ligated tissue slough away without cutting. Apply a bit of corrosive ointment to each site or apply a hot iron.

On occasion the hemorrhoid will not bleed but will drain pus. In such a case look to determine the direction in which to drain, either down toward the buttocks or into the anus. In the latter case you need do nothing. In the former, either insert a hot cautery (ie a stab) or use a corrosive ointment. Follow with the routine wound-care.

Addenda by Roland

A. Another remedy: Sorrel roots boiled in a fine white wine. Use it to fumigate the seated patient. This treatment dries and destroys the hemorrhoids. The smoke should be directed through a funnel.
B. The juice of pellitory, egg-yolk and oil of roses will decrease the swelling.

CHAPTER 50. STRANGURY AFTER WOUNDS

A suprapubic or perineal wound may cause strangury. We can offer some relief.

Make a plaster of the ashes of the leaves and the roots of elder trees boiled at length. Put some it in a sac and lay it over the pubis, as hot as tolerated. It will not delay urination.

CHAPTER 51. THE APPLICATION POINTS OF THE CAUTERY FROM THE SHOULDERS TO THE GROINS

Knowing the great benefits of the cautery everywhere in the body, I must comment here on the special therapeutic applications in the trunk, from the shoulders to the genitalia. We use them against swollen and inflamed joints in the hands and the arms and we use the arm to treat painful hands, and we apply it three finger-breadths away from a specific painful joint.

To treat inflammation and pain in a hand, burn in the dorsal hollow between the thumb and hand and in a web between two fingers on the other hand. To treat the upper arm, shoulders and eyes, burn the hollow at the elbow, both the inner and the outer surfaces. For asthma burn in the suprasternal notch. For liver disease burn directly over the organ

CHAPTER 52. SETONS

For splenic disorders, place a seton over the spleen. You may use two, placed well apart. For pain in the umbilicus, place one three fingerbreadths below.

For pain in the flank, place one in the lumbar hollow, and another three fingerbreadths below. For pain in the back, place two: one three fingerbreadths above, the other the same distance below.[76]

For pain in the testicles place a seton behind the scrotum, over the ischium.

For hemorrhoids place a seton above the anus.

HERE ENDS BOOK III OF THE CHIRURGIA

---

[76] The Seton Cautery was inserted through a fold of skin. When the track was charred, the seton was withdrawn and a probe with an 'eye' was inserted. The eye was threaded and the probe was withdrawn, leaving the thread in the channel. (LDR).

BOOK 1V

THE PELVIS AND LOWER EXTREMITIES

INTRODUCTION

Here I approach my goal to complete this work, with God's help. I know that my literary style is not elegant and my words are not colorful and my grammar is imperfect. I beg the forgiveness of my readers for those failures.

I hope that they will accept this work for what it is, a practical treatise. The order of presentation etc. are mine. But I have been constrained by it being firmly based (ie on Roger's work) on what deserves the praises of all men, and on his enduring fame.

So it is that here we follow his methods of dealing with matters affecting the pelvis and the lower extremities.

Chapter 1. Wounds Of The Hip And Pelvis

When a sword cuts at that level, remove all the loose matter and apply our medicines, according to whether or not you need sutures. If the weapon is a projectile and you cannot easily disimpact it, cut down on it to free it. If it is imbedded in bone you may use a trephine to drill holes around the metal head and then remove it. The usual medicines follow.

When the bone itself is not damaged, the treatment is simple.

Addendum by Roland

A. The vertebro (ie head of the femur) is included in the term 'hip', the pelvis.

Chapter 2. Wounds Of The Thigh

Cutting wounds of the thigh, with or without injury to the femur, are treated as we do for the arm.

The treatment of projectile wounds here is no different than in the arm.

CHAPTER 3 WOUNDS AT THE KNEE

Treat wounds which cut through the patella (or divide the quadriceps tendon) by suturing them. That holds also for all transverse cuts when the patella is not involved. If an arrowhead is lodged in the knee, remove it very carefully. Follow our procedures and our routines with medications

Addenda by Roland

A. We rarely see a complete recovery in these cases (ie without lameness).
B. In a case where the tendon between the thigh and the patella is cut we repair it by bandaging (ie holding the knee in extension). We may need to use a powder of rye-flour, mummy (or dry human blood if genuine mummy is not available) and sang-dragon. After grinding them add egg-white and apply it in the wound.

CHAPTER 4. WOUNDS OF THE LOWER LEG

For the most part use our usual methods. However, I should add this warning: When the wound occurs within three inches above or below the knee and involves more than just muscle, be aware of the fearful consequences.[77] When you treat those wounds with our ordinary measures and you observe swelling, induration and dark discoloration which spreads proximally, the outcome will be fatal.

Penetrating wounds caused by projectiles call for our routine methods.

CHAPTER 5. WOUNDS OF THE FEET

Treat all these wounds, including those which affect the nerves and the bones, as we treated hand-wounds.

---

[77] See Fn.57, Bk. II, Ch.10. and Fn.58, Bk.II, Ch.11.(LDR)

If the calcaneus is damaged, you must exercise special attention and care (ie as to the length of the leg).

Chapter 6. Dislocated Hip

When a great fall or a severe blow causes a dislocated hip and a collection of humors in the joint and the nerves (ie tendons and ligaments as well as nerves) are torn, the damage is a permanent limp, although some improvement can be obtained.

Place the patient flat on his back. The surgeon sits facing him, pulling the lower leg, while a robust assistant pulls the body cephalad. The surgeon manipulates the leg while applying traction below and pushing the femoral head with a foot below the groin to replace it. The patient helps by rolling while the measurements are made from the buttock-creases to the heels. When they are the same, all is well.

Then lay on a moist (egg-white) cloth and pads where needed, and enclose them with a bandage that pulls the thighs and hips together . Put the patient supine in a narrow cot which will restrict his movements. Anoint and foment him frequently with our familiar medicines.

Chapter 7. Fractures Of The Femur

When the femur is fractured, first realign the fragments. If in addition there is an open wound, distract the fragments and bit-by-bit fit the exposed ends together. Then treat the wound as you did for fractures of the humerus. Always compare the injured side with the normal so that the feet, the legs and the thighs all match. Leave a gap of about the width of one finger-nail between the bone ends.[78]

---

[78] The Latin word 'uncia' is translated, either as one inch or one finger-nail-width in different texts. The reason for leaving such a gap between the ends of the fragments in a realigned fracture is not explained. Perhaps the surgeon anticipated that the bone-ends would settle against each other or that callus would bridge the gap. The later authors ignore the recommendation (LDR).

When you bind on the splints extend them beyond the fracture, equidistant above and below. If there is an open wound, do not cover it, as we have taught.

Chapter 8. Dislocations At The Hip And Knee

We treat here just as we do for dislocations at the shoulder and the elbow. First we use inunctions and fomentations and then with a stirrup-strap we produce a sudden strong force to reduce the displaced femur. Then we bind the limb, first in flexion and then in extension, without the use of splints. Then gradually we rehabilitate with a schedule of ambulatory exercises.

Chapter 9. Fractures Of The Leg With And Without Open Wounds

Here we follow the methods we used for fractures of the humerus, with this exception, already noted for fractures of the femur; we leave a gap of one finger-nail breadth between the proximal and distal fragments and we use splints and bindings. Remember this as well: a fracture of the tibia or of the femur within three inches of the knee which produces the ominous signs we have described threatens the life of the victim.

Chapter 10. Dislocations Of The Ankle And Toes

A foot may be dislocated at the ankle and it may dangle medially or laterally, or it may be dorsiflexed or bent downward. In this case we first use our usual fomentations and inunctions. Then the surgeon applies strong traction on the foot and restores the normal position, according to the case. Then he sets suitable splints and binds them in place.

When a toe is displaced we reduce it just as we did a dislocated finger.

Chapter 11. Cancers and Fistulas In The Above Regions

As a consequence of the above cancers and fistulas (ie chronic ulcers) may occur in the soft tissues.[79] Or, the result may be an infected or infarcted (ie carious) bone. The former can be treated safely by ablation with the actual or with virtual cauteries (ie corrosives), [80] because the region is devoid of nerves, arteries and veins. However, this kind of cancer may be localized or it may spread. When you use the actual cautery to treat the spreading cancer (ie gangrene) extend your burn at the margins and in depth until you reach tissues which bleed. Then medicate with eggs and the other substances that we use.

When the bony lesion is localized and shows itself as a protrusion pointing through the overlying intact skin, apply a waxen or pasty capsule of corrosive materials to fit directly over the mass and cover the surrounding healthy skin with wax or paste to protect it from the corrosives. Reapply the corrosives until the damaged bone is exposed. Leave on the capsule all day or overnight and then apply eggs to mitigate the inflammation and pain caused by the corrosives.

When the overlying skin is eaten away and you can see the bony lesion (ie active osteomyelitis or a sequestrum), get rid of the bad part—the black, dead and infected matter—with a rasp, as used by the hand of an experienced surgeon. The exposed healthy tissues will grow to cover the bone, as it does in cases treated with the actual cautery.

If the gangrene in the bone is too extensive, the case is incurable. You may provide some relief by controlling the spread at the margins with strong depilatories. The malodorous tissues can be destroyed with a powder of asphodels.

---

[79] See Fn. 64, Bk.III, Ch. 22 (LDR).

[80] The disease bone is then scraped away (LDR).

Addendum by Roland

A. In the leg, over the shin, a lupus may form. This differs from cancers in ways we have described. In such a case we incise three
finger-breadths (ie proximal) and undermine the lupus and cut
the roots, bit-by-bit. Then we apply oakum with egg-yolk.[81]

The following day we cauterize (ie cut away the ulcer) with care
and apply powders and ointments as we do for cancers (ie gangrenous ulcers).

Chapter 12. Pustules And Lacerations In The Leg

We treat them much as we did in the head. In addition: We begin
by thoroughly washing the leg with the patients own urine, voided
that morning. Then we dry the leg well before applying the recommended ointments. When we observe progress toward healing, we
change to the white ointment made with rose-water and oil of violets
in place of vinegar and common oil.

Chapter 13. Where To Apply The Cautery In The Lower Extremity

For sciatica, touch the pointed cautery in three places above the
trochanter or use a triangular cautery.

For treating disorders of the torso: burn three times in the leg: 1.
Three fingerbreadths below the knee; 2. Three fingerbreadths above
the medial malleolus (this is very effective in treating arthritis and
pains in the upper body); 3. Anywhere over the calf.

For arthritis, burn deep (ie puncture) the soles of the feet.

---

[81] This is a fair description of a treatment for a venous stasis ulcer by interrupting
the underlying 'feeder' veins (LDR).

Chapter 14. Burns Cause By Flames Or Boiling Water

When treating these burns first wash throroughly with an emulsion of common oil and cold water, adding the cold water while you shake the mixture. Then anoint the burn.

Another remedy: Pomegranate bark steeped in a fine wine for a long time before bringing it to a boil. Remove and grind the bark with egg-white and use it as an ointment.

Another: Take a handful each of the cold herbs (ie crassula major and minor) , dill, penny-wort, solathrum and leeks. Mash them with one pound of fresh lard. Heat all in a sauce-pan and filter before adding wax and some mastic. This is a good medicine.

Another: Take elder-tree twigs and crush them a little and then mix in some lard. Let it stand for three days and then boil the lot in water. Filter it and save the filtrate for use.

Chapter 15. Deep And Penetrating Inflammations

Use this ointment to treat such: Take one ounce each of litharge and burnt lead, five ounces each of mastic and olibanum and four ounces of walnut kernels. Grind all to a powder. Then take the juice mashed from three ounces each of stone-crop, umbellicus venus,. solathrum and blackberry twigs and take three ounces of oil of violets. Shake the oil with the juices and mix in the powder.

Another topical: Add rose-water to the white ointment and spread it on a leaf of plantain or cabbage which you lay on the inflamed part.

Another: Quick-lime stirred in water. Shake it well and let the lime settle. Decant and discard the water. Repeat the wash three times. Then take some oil of violets, oil of roses and common oil and mix them with the lime residue and shake well with some added water. Save the oily part for use.

An effective remedy is saracenic soap which is made according to strict rules (ie see below) and mixed with honey to make a topical.

Addenda by Roland

A. Another remedy: Take alum, vinegar and honeysuckle. The mixture will relieve pain in a short time. The same relief may be obtained with pigeon droppings (ie a paste). Another: common oil, oil of roses and oil of violets, mix and apply on the burns and follow with a powder of incinerated donkey turds.

B. Make Saracenic soap this way: Take two measures of potash lye and one of common oil and simmer them until they thicken, such that droplet does not spread on a marble tile or when a tiny bit placed on the tongue does not sour and cause burning. Then add a third measure if the lye and cook until the thickness is correct, as tested on the marble; the tongue will feel only a hint of a 'bite'. Again add two measures of lye and repeat the actions. Now the perfect density will be indicated by the droplet and by a benign effect on the tongue. The product will be dark; hence the name is Saracenic (ie dark-skinned).

CHAPTER 16. THE VARIETIES OF LEPROSY AND THEIR TREATMENTS[82]

The excesses of four humors cause all four types of leprosy: alopecia,. elephantiasis, leontiasis and psoriatiasis (ie teriasis).

Alopecia derives from phlegm and has reference to foxes.[83] Elephantiasis is caused by sanguinous humors and has a name which refers to enlargement, indirectly relating it to the largest animal as well as to the most profuse humor, which is blood. Leontiasis derives from natural bile. The name indicates its lion-like qualities: heat refers to the hottest of the animals, the lion, and to the lion's various colors seen in this kind of leprosy. The psoriatic leprosy comes from black bile and the name

---

[82] Leprosy was a waste-basket diagnosis, as one sees it here. Baldness and alopecia areata, lymphedema of any source and ulcerated pruritic dermatoses were included. Probably the deformities and the facies of leontiasis were the only manifestations of leprosy as we name it, although no mention is made of that notorious facial manifestation (LDR).

[83] The Greek word for fox is alwphx. Foxes shed their winter fur in clumps, hence alopecia areata (LDR.

refers to the suffering cause by the intense itching which makes the victim rub and tear at his clothing (ie Latin 'terere' to rub) as he interminably seeks relief. For relief in that case we use this ointment: Take four ounces of French soap, one pound of pitch, three ounces each of wax and borax, four ounces each lupine-flour and soot (ie lamp-black), three ounces of the juice of fumitory, four ounces of old lard and sufficient amounts of oil and potash-lye. Mix the ingredients (excepting those which first have to be ground to powders) in an earthenware pot and heat them to liquefy them before adding the wax to what you have powdered. Use it warm and apply it daily for a week. Then bathe the patient to remove the accumulated ointment. After three daily baths, amputate his testicles and apply a cautery (ie a point application) in the hollow of the elbow where the humerus ends, and on both ears, at the special points (designated for leprosy). This ointment also may be useful for elephantiasis.

For alopecia you also may use this: Take four ounces each of pepper and live sulfur, three ounces of pyrethrum and one small jug (ie amphora) filled with oil and another filled with garlic-juice and one pound of French soap. Pulverize the solids and mix them in the boiling oils. Add the soap while stirring over the fire. Shave away the remaining fuzz (ie lanugo in the bald areas) and then vigorously rub the surfaces with wool. Follow that with a sweat bath and a dry interval when you anoint the patient. Repeat the treatment every three days until normal hair growth persists (ie instead of lanugo).

Chapter 17. Spasm After Wounds [84]

Treat spasms which complicate wounds as follows: First anoint the patient with the Greek ointment, made so: Take one ounce of the oil of musk, five ounces of petroleum (ie probably crude oil), four ounces each of common oil and butter, one ounce of wax, two drams each of styrax, calamite and madder, five ounces each of mastic and olibanum, three drams of gum-arabic and clematis. Mix everything (excepting the powders) and heat it until it is liquid. Then add the powders as you stir with a spatula. Add the styrax last when the liquidity is just right. Put the liquid on the three anti spasm points (on the nape, on the throat and over the spine) Then you may spread some of it over the body. The medicine is effective against all spasms cause by plethora.

Addendum by Roland

A. Another remedy: Take a handful each of absinthe, laurel berries and cinnamon. Grind them and add honey. Bring it to a boil to thicken it. Spread it on a napkin and apply that on the painful part. It is a wonderful analgesic.

HERE ENDS THE CHIRURGIA OF MASTER ROGER

---

[84] The term remains unexplained here. Certainly, tetanus was one kind of 'spasm' of concern to the surgeon. The Arabic and Classical authors give it full attention and the medieval authors who followed Roger dealt with it at length.

Perhaps we should remind ourselves after we have read Roger's book, as scanty and as limited in scope we may have found it, that he had few sources on which to lean when he set out to revive his art. The translations of the Arabic texts were just then coming into the hands of a chosen few Europeans. We do Roger an injustice to compare him with the great Albucasis whose finely written texts were more available to the leading surgeons during the century after Roger. After all, we must consider Albucasis himself, a century and half before Roger, the acme of Arabic surgery, as a copyist of his own near and distant predecessors. Much of what we read read in Roger's Chirurgia was derived from the experiences of an ingenious and observant surgeon who also was a willing teacher, esteemed by the pupils who wrote this treatise. (LDR).

A COMPENDIUM PHARMACOPEIA
OF MEDIEVAL SURGICAL MEDICATIONS

INTRODUCTION

Our texts of Roger's Chirurgia contain no pharmacopeias as such, although Hunt added a fine glossary of Anglo-Norman terms to assist the readers of his edition. Therein they will find that many of the medications mentioned in his Ms. differ in names and applications from what we find in the other texts.

Therefore, I have appended a compendium pharmacopeia which contains nearly all of the medical substances used by Roger (including those from Hunt) and the other seven great surgeons who wrote their treatises during the century and half after him. I have culled the list from the texts available to me. The Rogerine Latin Ms and the Italian translations of it contain the commentaries (ie Addenda) of Roland, and I have placed his list with Roger's. I have not gone to another source for Roland, who admitted with pride that his book was simply a revised edition of the Rogerina.

THE FORMAT

The list is alphabetical. The numbered and lettered items are from my English texts of William of Saliceto, Lanfranchi of Milan and Henri de Mondeville, where they refer to the substances in the antidotaries that are parts of their works. The medicines used by Roger Frugard, Bruno of Longoburgo, Theodoric of Cervia and Jehan of Ypres are not numbered, except as they are included as users of the numbered items, which are in the majority.

Following each entry there are synonyms, one or more common names and variant spellings, and the names which modern translators have used in the Italian and Anglo-Norman French editions of Roger (**R**)—and Roland , the Italian of Bruno (**B**), The English of Theodoric (**T**), the French of William (**W**), Henri (**H**), and Yperman (**Y**) and the Middle-English of Lanfranchi (**L**). Those initials in bold-face type at the end of most of the entries indicate the authors who mentioned the substances which I have culled from the texts that were available to me. Many of the items are followed by "see" which refer the reader to numbered items for additional information.

Wherever I can do so, I identify the plants by more recent botanical terms. I cannot claim accuracy in many cases, especially where the 19thC and 20thC botanists and herbalists have themselves confused me with contrary nomenclatures. I have used Professor Saint-Lager's terminology in Henri de Mondeville's text and Mrs. Grieve's book as well as dictionaries and encyclopedias for assistance in those matters. The Alphita has helped in some cases.

As stated above in the Introduction, I believe that there are only a few items missing from the following, and I apologize for any such deficienies. The list probably is a nearly complete surgical pharmacopeia for the century and half spanned by the major written works of the epoch.

THE LIST

1. Absinthe — oil of wormwood, avrotonin, aloisne. *Artemesia (sev.species)*. **R B W L H Y**

Abrotonin — see 35

2. Acacia — prunella juice (not the plum tree). *Prunella spinosa.*. **B T W L H**

3. Acanthus — Bear's breech. see 64. *Acanthus mollis.* **L**

4. Ache — see 29, 97. *Apium graveolum.*. **R W L**

Acedula — see 395. **H**

Acetosa — see 484. also *Rumex acetosa.* see 395. **R W L H**

5. Acoris — sweet sedge. see 74, 75, 408, 422, 434, 444. **R W L**

Acorns — glans quercus. see 203, 309a. **H**

6. Acus muscata — Robert's herb, crispula, geranium. see 366. *Geranium Robertianum.* **H**

7. Adiantum — delicate ferns, maiden hair, venus hair. see 363. *Adiantum capillus veneris.* **T W**

Adeps — see 206. **W L H**

8. Adracanth — see 466. **Y**

9. Adustum — see 38. **L**

10. Aes — chalcanthum, ios, bronze. **W L H**

Affodil — see 40, 43, and sometimes 301. **R W**

11. Agaric — a mushroom. *Polyporus igniarius.* **R T W H**

Agnus castus — see 205. also chaste-tree, *Vitex trifolia.* **T**

12. Agresta — sour-grape (uva acerba) juice, celidonia, verjus; (also memitte, a poppy). see 335, 478. *Vitri vinifera.* **T L H**

13. Agrimony	St. John's Herb. see 172. *Agrimonia eupatorium.* **R T H**
Ailes	allium. see 43. **W**
14. Airaine	'flower' of bronze, areim, ereim, eneim. see 481. **R W L H**
Alabaster	see 214. **Y**
Albugasse	see 286. **W**
Alexander's Ivy	see 256. **T**
15. Alkanna	henna *Lawsonia inermis.* **T W H**
16. Alleluia	a clover, weed sorrel, oxalis, paniscuculi. see 395. **R L H**
Allium	see 43a, 278a. **R H**
17. Almonds	bitter or sweet. *Amygdalis communis.* **W H**
18. Althea	guimauve, geumalve, marsh mallow, bismalve. see 273. **R B T W L H**
19. Aloes	aloe vera, picra, pigré. Horse aloes are unpurified. *Aloe socotrina..* **R B T W L H Y**
20. Alum (alun)	from wine lees (potassium tartrate) or from crystals. (alun de roche is sugar-alum, aluminum sulfate, alumen de pluma (feather alum) is halotrichite, iron-aluminum sulfate) etc.. **R B T W L H**
Amber	see 85. **T W H**
Ambrosia	balsameta, herb St.Mary. see 49, 200 **R**
21. Amidum	flour of various grains, amylum, usually wheat, froment. see 177, 436, 494. **T W L H Y**
22. Ammi	seeds. see 205. **W**
23. Ammoniaque	hore-hound. resin of *Dorema ammoniacum.* or *Bubon gummifer.* **B W L H Y**
24. Amome	ginger family. see 201. **W**
24a. Amorantus	almarus, amens *Amaranthus hypochondria.* **T**
Anabulle	see 173. **H**
25. Anacardus	cashew nuts, elephant's foot. *Semicarpus anacordium.* **T W L H**
Anagallis	see 93.

25a. Andronium   a primrose. *Primula vulgare.* **T**

25b. Anemone   wind-flower and herb. *Anemone pulsatella.* **T**

26. Aneth   dill, or sweet anise, siler, sifula see 158. *Anethum graveolens.* **R W L H**

26a. Angelica   emperor's herb. see 167. *Angelica archangelica.* **W H**

27. Anise   leaves and seeds. see 349. *Pimpinelle anisum.* **R W H Y**

     Annaglossa   see 353.

     Anthera   see 389. **H**

28. Antimony   stibium, metal filings. **T W L H Y**

28a. Ants   insects and eggs. **T L**

28b.Apis   honey bee. **H**

29. Apium   many species. ache, batrachium, patalupi, wild celery. see 4. *Apium graveolens.* **T W L H**

30. Apostolicon   Apostles' Ointment from twelve ingredients: 23, 33, 53, 188, 194, 253, 299, 312, 321, 379, 482, 493 also called Black Ointment and Venus ointments. **R B T W L H Y**

30a. Apricot   *Prunus armenica.* **T**

     Apozym   a decoction of various roots.

     Apple   see 363a.

30b. Aqua   forte nitric acid. **W**

31. Araignee   spider web. **R**

31a. Argentum Vivum mercury. see 383. **W H Y**

31b. Arancium   see 119, 322. **W L**

32. Argilla   terra sigulina. clay. **W L H**

33. Aristolochium   snake-root, malum terrae, polyrrhyzon, clematis, birth-wort. see 58, 120, 142, 376. *Aristolochium rotunda.* **R T W L H Y**

     Armoniacum   armenian apricots. see 23, 30a. *Prunus armeniacus.* **R T W** (or Sal armoniacus. see 424.)

34. Arsenic   auripigmentum, sublimate of arsenic sulfate. see 327. **R B T W L H Y**

35. Artimesa   a(b)vrotonon, citronella, mugwort, armoise, avrone salvage, St. John's plant, absinthe. *Artemisia vulgare.* **R W L H**

35a. Arum	dracuntium minus, serpentaria, cuckoo-pint, dracunculus. *Dracunculus vulgaris.* **T H**
Arundo	see 386. **W**
36. Asa Dulcis	sweet gum, laser, benzoin, tapsii. see 461. *Styrax benzoin* . **T W**
37. Asafoetida	assa *Ferula foetida.* **B T W L H**
37a. Asclepias	milkweed. *sev.Asclepiadaceae* **R**
38. Ashes	see 60, 98, 101, 106, 111, 115. **R B T W H**
Ash tree	see 189, 264. **H**
Aspen tree	see 364a. **H**
39. Asperge	asparagus roots or stems. *Asparagus officinalis.* **T H**
40. Asphodel	albutum, affodil, anthericon, centum capitum, porrago. roots of *Asphodelus albus.* **R W L H**
41. Assefan	styrax. see 36, 447. **W**
41a. Assius lapis	a stone from Assa (the Troad). **W**
Atrement	atrament. vitriol based. see 490. **W Y**
42. Atriplex hortense	orache, arroche, pes locustae. *Atriplex hortensis.* **T W H**
43. Aulx	ailes, garlic, allium, elinnium, affodile (wild), ramsome, porrum. *Allium sativum.* **R T W L**
43a. Aunée	scabwort, inula. spikenard. see 437. *Inula helenium.* **T W**
43b. Aurea	aurum. a decoction of gold particles in water or vinegar. **T**
43c. Auripigmentum.	see 34, 327. **R T W L H**
Avellana	hazel nuts. see 134a, 309. **R.**
Avena	haveron. see 310. **T H**
Avrotonin	abrotinin. see 35. **T W L**
44. Axonge	lard, lardon, oint, sui, axungia. see 206. **R L H Y**
45. Bacca populi	poplar berries, bourgeon. see 364a. **W**
46. Baccar	asarum, asarabacca. *Asarum europaeum.* **W**
47. Balaustium	wild pomegranate flowers. see 364. **R B W L H Y**
48. Balsamdendron	balm of gilead, xylobalsamum. see 53, 90. *Balsamodendron opobalsamum.* **T W H**

49. Balsameta	St. Mary's herb, costmary, mace, ambrosia, chenopodium. *Tamacetum balsamita.* **R H**
49a. Barba hircina	salsify, goat's beard. *Tragopogon porrifolius.* **W**
49b. Bardana	see 236 and 395 (also Burdock, arctium lappa). **R H**
50. Barecha	see 280, 369. **W**
50a. Basilicon Oint.	53, 206, 312, 360, 379, 493. see 314. **H**
51. Basilium	basilicon, herb basil, wall-thyme. *Ocymum basilicum.* **T W H**
Battitura	see 106. **T**
52. Baucia	pastinaca. parsnip or carrot. see 152. **L H**
53. Bdellium	procerion. a balsamic resin. see 48. *Balsamodendron africanum.* **T W L H Y**
53a Bedagar	wild roses, eglantiere. **R?**
Beans	see 178. **T**
Belladonna	see 217.
53a. Belliculus	blata bysantia, belliculli marini. purple and white marine snails, source of royal purple dye. **T W**
Belsegensina	see 132. **W**
53b. Ben	been. *Moringa aptera* .**W**
53c. Bendegard	bedegar. gall from stem of eglantine rose. see 389. **W**
Bennett	Herb Bennett. see 115, 116.
54. Beta	Bleta , betta, beets. *Chenopodiacia.* **W H**
55. Berberis	mountain grape, cortex bugia. see 68. *Berberis vulgaris.* **L H**
55a. Berula	an herb. *Berula angustifolia.* **T H**
56. Betonica	betony, scrofularia, figwort, vetony. see 155a. *Betonica officinalis.* **R T H**
57. Bile	melanchiron, fiel, fellis. see 183. **B T W L H**
58. Birthwort	asirinum, aristolochium, snake root. see 33. **T**
Black Ointment	see 30. **Y**
58a. Blackberry	see 393. **Y**
Blood	see 409.

59. Bol d'armenie   a clay containing iron oxide, various clays—German, Bohemian, etc.-sometimes fuller's earth, cimoleam. **R B T W L H Y**

60. Bombacyna   see 107, 333. etc. **T W**

61. Bone-marrow   medulla, midolle, meule. see 275. **T H**

62. Bones   of geese or hens, hooves, ivory, squid etc., all burned and powdered. **R T W L H**

63. Borax   borax, sodium borate; see sal de nitre, also sagimen nitri, nitrum, boracis, bourac. **R W L H Y**

63a. Borrago   bourache, borrage. see 69. **R T L H**

63b. Boxwood   dogwood, ammon's horn. *Cornus amonum and floridum.* **T**

Bran   see 21. **T**

64. Branca Ursina   acanthus, brama, bear's brush. see 3. *Acanthus mollis or Heraclium spondylum.* **T L H**

64a. Brassica   generic term. see 71, 377 et al.

65. Bread   crumbs are mica panis, see 285. **T W L.** Panata is a bread soup. **W** Opirus is whole-wheat bread. **T**

Bronze   see 14.

66. Broom   planta genesta. *Cytisus scoparius.* **H**

Brown Ointment   a regenerative mentioned only by referral to Nicholas.

Bruscus   butcher's broom. see 221, 226a. *Ruscus aculatis.* **R T W**

67. Bryonia   brionee, viticelle, root of bryony, also sicadis, labrusca. see 120, 182, 489. *Bryonia dioecia.* (White bryony, a poison, is *Momordica elaterum*, really a cucumber). **R T W L H**

68. Bugia   root-bark of barberry bush, cortex bugia. see 55. **W H**

69. Bugloss   borrago, blue weed, lingua bovis, lange de boef. see 416. *Borrago officianalis or Anchusa officianalis..* **R T W L H**

Bulbus	see 319, 415. **W**
Burdock	see 236 and 395. **R**
Burith	see 412. **R**
70. Butter	from cows, also sweet butter, May butter, bure de mai. **B T W L H**
71. Cabbage	choux, chaux, caulis, cholet, cavolo. *Brassica oleracea.* **R T W L H**
Cacumia	see 121. **W**
72. Calamint	see thyme. *Melissa calaminthus.* **T W H**
73. Calamite	styrax. see 447. **T W**
74. Calamus	aromaticus, squinanthus, sweet sedge, sweet flag. see 5, 75, 444. **B T W L Y**
Calx viva	quick-lime. see 251. **L H Y**
Camedreos	see 200.
75. Camel grass	see 74, 416a, 422, 444. *Andropogon schoenanthus.* **H**
76. Camomille	chamomile (several varieties) cotula. *Anthemis nobilis and A. pyrethrum.* **B T W L H Y**
76a. Campanula	rampion. *Campanula indicas.* **T**
77. Camphor	champhore, caphura. *Laurus camphora.* **R T W L H Y**
78. Cannabis	hemp seeds or leaves, chévenis. *Cannabis sativa.* **H Y**
Canne	see 378a and 386. **T W**
79. Cannelle	cinnamon. *Laurus cinnamomum.* **R H Y**
80. Cantharides	spanish fly. Eloe vesicatorum. **B T L H**
81. Capers	capparis. fruits, shells, bark, oil. lonacera, a honeysuckle. *Capparis spinosa.* **R T W H**
Capillus veneris	see 7. **H**
82. Capital Powder	19, 33,188 228, 299, 325, 329, 408, 410. For head-wounds. **T H Y**
83. Capitellum	capiteils, potash lye, lessive. see 254. **R L H**
Capreoli	see 208.
84. Caprifolium	caprifici, cheirefoile, honeysuckle, licius. a fig. see 260. *Lonicera caprifolium.* **R H**

85. Carabe   amber, possibly containing a scarab beetle. **W H**
86. Cardamom   amomie, granum paradisis, granum solis. *Amimum cardamomum.* **T L H Y**
    Cardo   see 102.**R H Y**
87. Carmingella   an aromatic herb, unidentified
88. Carnis serpentum snake meat. see 129. **H**
89. Carolus   dry-rot wood of fallen trees. **W**
90. Carpobalsama   see 49. **W H**
    Carrot   see 52, 152. **T**
91. Carthame   safflowers and seeds. see 298. *Carthamus tinctorius.* **R W**
92 Carvum   caraway seeds. *Carum carvi.* **T W**
93. Caryophyla   garyophyla, giroflé, sanamunda, herb-benedict, cloves, eugenia, anagallus, carnations, chickweed, stellaria, ipia. see 155a, 202. *Caryophylus aromaticus or Geum urbanum.* **B T W L H**
    Cashew   see 25.
94. Cassia 'bastard' cinnamon. and many others. see 427 *Laurus cassia.* **T W L H Y**
    Cassilago   see 217. **R H**
95. Castor bean   ricinus, cataputia, cocconidium. Diacastor is a laxative electuary. *Ricinus communis.* **B T W H Y**
96. Castoreum   beaver musk. **R B H**
96a Cathimia   cadmia, lapis calaminaris. see 121, 439. **T H**
    Cauda equina   hippuris see 170. **W H**
    Caul   see 71. **W H**
96a. Cedar tree   of Lebanon. *Cedrus libani.*
97. Celery (wild)   see 4.
98. Celandine   chelidoine (probably the 'lesser'), figwort;. see 56, 109. **T**
99. Cendre de chêne   ashes of Turkish oak (Quercus cerris) lexivium, see 117, 254.

100 Centaurée	jacea, narce. thistle, see teazle. **T W L H**
Centinervia	see 428. **R**
Centrum	galli gallitricum. See 196
101. Cepa	oignun, ascalonia. onion. see 229, 243, 319. **W L H**
101a. Ceratonus	any of four legumes including carob. **W**
102. Cerdone	cardo, chardun, calendula, thistle, senecio. see 100, 458. *Centauria centaurium or Cardo benedictus.* **R H**
103. Cerebrum galli	chicken brain. **H**
104. Cerisier	cerice, cherry tree, bark, sap. *Prunus avium.* **R L**
105. Ceruse	white lead, psimythion, minium. see 242. **R T W L H Y**
Ceterach	see 438a. **T H**
106. Chalcécaumené	chalcanthum. copper sulfate and other metallic salts, battitura see 481, 482. **T W L H Y**
Chalmedrys	kamedrys. see 200. **W**
107. Charte de soit	bombacyna, papyrus. ashes of paper made from silk. see 38,107 333. **W**
Chaux	calx. see 251. **T W L H Y**
108. Chebules	kebuklus. see 298 (unripe). **T W L H Y**
109. Chelidonium	celidoine salvage, celandine. see 12, 98. *Chelidonium majus or Ficaria ranunculoidis.* **W L H**
Chenopodium	see 49
Cherry	see 104
110. Chestnut	nux castanearum, chastaine. see 309. *Castanea sativa.* **R T L**
111. Cheveux humaine	ashes from human hair, capillae humani. see 117. **T**
112. Chick peas	cicer. *Cicer arietinum.* **T W L H**
Chick-weed	see 445a.
113. Chicory	leaves. also endives, scariola. *Cichorium intybus.* **L**
China root	see 193.

113a. Cicada	incinerated insect. **T**
Cicer	see 112. **H**
114. Ciclamen	pome de terre, malum terrae, sowbread, cyclamen, earth-nut, panis porcinus. see 33, 262. *Conopodium majus or Cyclamen hederifolium.* **R L H**
115. Cicuta	cowbane, water hemlock, cicuta virosa, benedicta. see 116. *Conium maculatum.* **R L H**
116. Ciguë	hemlock seeds, herb bennet, beneite. see 115. *Conium maculatum..* **R H**
Cimolea	cymolia. see 289. **H**
117. Cinis	various woods, bones, crabs, mouse, rabbit, scorpion, sponge, hair, grapevine, oyster shell, seashells, seashell, hair, paper, etc. see 38. **T W L H**
Cinnabar	minium. see 241. **W**
117a. Cinnamon	see 79. **T W H Y**
Cinq-foil	tormentilla. see 465. **T H**
118. Cissus	cissus, hedera, Virginia creeper. *Vitis hederacea.* **H**
Cistus	see 234
Citonia	and oil. see 185. **W**
119. Citrons	cedrovarious citrus fruits and melons. Venarum citrinum is citrus fruit pulp. see 31b, 250. **B W H**
Citrouilles	gourds, melons. see 280. **R T W H**
120. Clematis	the flower, ground-ivy, iere, viticella, vitis petit vigne, hedera, flammula, aristolochium. see 33, 376. *Clematis vitalis and Hedera helix, etc.* **R T L H**
121. Climie argenti	metallic oxides, espec. zinc, also cacumia, cathimia, spode, tuthie, silver, iron, couperose. **T W L H**
122. Clove	see 93.

122a Clover	various trifoils, perhaps flaura. see 191, 277. *Trifolium pratensa.* **T**
Cochia	a laxative compound pill, hierarufinum. see 125. **T**
122b. Coctana	dwarf figs. see 185. **W**
123. Coing	quince. citonium, diacydomite. see 372. **W**
123a. Cold Seeds	'cold-weather seeds'. The Greater are 137, 144, 192, 280. The Lesser are 245, 368, 392. see 423. **T W**
124. Colle	gelatin ('gluten'). Vellis vaccini is cowhide as a source. see 204, 368a, 431a. **H**
124a.Colchicum	see 141, 219. **Y**
Colcothar	see 490. **T W H**
125. Colocynth	"bitter apple' or bitter cucumber, cucurbite. see 67 see cocchia. *Cucumis colocynthis.* **W L H**
126. Colophony	see 352. **R B T W L H Y**
127. Columbine	culver-wort, sparagus, geranium molle, pigeon foot. *Geranium columbinum.* **B T**.
Comfrey	see 128. **R T H Y**
127a. Condisicale	condes. Not identified, perhaps an ointment based on rye flour. see 395a. **T**
128. Consoude	comfrey, consolida, greinure. *Symphytum officinalis (large) or Brunella vulgare (small).* **R B T W L H Y**
Convolvulus	see 416
129. Cooked meats	beef, lamb, pork, veal, snake, frog and various domestic and wild fowls, and their organs. Sometimes the specifiied source was a castrated male animal. **T W L**
130. Copper	calchanthum. see 106, 482, etc. **T W L H Y**
131. Corail	coral polyps(red and white), sponge stone. see 162. **W L H**
132. Coriander herb	belsegensima. *Coriander sativum.* **T W H**
Corigiola	see 361. **L H**.
133. Cornu	powdered horns of deer and goats, etc. **L H**

134. Cortex pini	bark of pine tree. see 350. *Pinus sylvestris.* **T L H**
134a. Coriolus	hazel tree. *Corylus genus.* **R**
135. Coste	various roots and oils including *Costus arabicus.* **T W H**
Cotonia	and cotonea malum. see 372. **L H**
136a. Coudrier.	hazel. see 215a. **Y**
136. Cotyledon	umbellicus venus, wall pennyroyal. see 420. **L H**
Couperose	see 106, 482, 490. **L H Y**
137. Courges	zucchini. Juices are elacterina. see 144a. *Cucurbita maxima.* **W**
138. Crab (river)	cancer fluvialis, granchia titrata, crab-meat and shells. **B L**
139. Crassula	major and minor, sedum, stonecrop, orpine, andrachne, mamilla muris, tegularia, vermicularis. *Sedum purpurascens.* **R L H**
Creta marina	chalk. see 251. **T H**
140. Crisomel	oil from orange seeds. **W**
140a Crithimum	samphire, St. Peter's herb, cretani. *Crithimum maritimum.* **T**
141. Crocus	saffron. see 124a, 219. **W L H**
142. Crows' feet	pes corvus, pes milvi. see 33, 120, 376. *Ranunculus sceleratus.* **T W L**
143. Cubebs	a pepper. *Piper cubeba..* **W L Y**
144. Cucumber	cultivated or wild, momordique, cucumiscelle. *Cucumis var.* **R W L H**
144a Cucurbite	melons, watermelon is cocomera. see 137. Many species. **R W L**
145. Cumin	comin, the herb *Cumin cyminum.* **R W Y**
146. Curcuma	turmeric. see 503. *Curcuma longa.* **T L H**
147. Currants	fresh or dried.
148 Cuscuta'	dodder; see 169.**R T**
Cuttle-fish bone	squid. see 62
Cylotrum	an arsenical and lime corrosive. see 327. **Y**

148a.Cynoglossus	cinoglossus, hound's-tongue herb, leaves and roots.
148b. Cyperes succus	a sedge. see 422. The nuts are from *C. Sempervirem*. **B W L H**
149. Cyprés	the tree.cypress nuts (seeds), bark, leaves and berries. see 396 . *Cyperus longus, C. rotundus*. **R B W L H Y**
150. Dactylus	dates of palm *Phoenix dactilifera*. Diaphoenicon is a laxative electuary of dates. **R T W H**
Daffodil	roots and flowers. see 301. **T**
151. Damascus plums	see 355
152. Daucus	carrot, baucia. *Daucius carota*. **R T H**
Delphinium	see 445.
152a Dentale	lead-wort. *Plumbago europaea'*. **T**
153. Diachylon	Mesüe's (one of several versions, see 284a.) ointment made of: 18, 26, 76, 124, 181, 185, 206, 228, 252, 253, 311, 379, 443, 459, 493. **T**
Diagridum	see 416 **W**
154. Diamargaritum	rubis troscicata, troche based on 342 and 393. **W Y**
155. Diamoron	a syrup of 294. see 317a. **W**
155a. Dianthus	a betony (56) and an electuary based on 387. **T**
Diaphoenicon	see 150
156. Diarhodon	an astringent powder from 2, 27, 59, 116, 407 (3 kinds), 460. **W**
Diatesseron	see 462. **T**
157. Diazinziber	a purgative made from 79, 86, 93, 201, 276,2 95. **W**
158. Dill	leaves and seeds. see 26. **R B**
159. Dipsaccus	teazle thistle, carduus, cardo.see 458, 487. *Cardo fullonum and Dipsaccus sylvestris*. **L H**
Dock	see 395.
160. Dodder	see 148, 169. Hell weed, (lesser dodder).

Dogwood	corneola,oil. see 63b. **R T H**
160a. Dove's Dung	star of Bethlehem. *Ornothogalum umbellatum.* **T**
160b. Dove's Foot	sparagi, *Geranium Molle.* **R**
161. Dragantum	iron peroxide, calcantum, colcothar chalcidis. see 490. sometimes 466. **R T L H**
161a.Dragon-weed	tarragon. Dracunculus vulgaris. **T**
Earthworms	see 258 and 499.
Ebulus	see 165 and 406. **R H**
162. Écume de Mer	meerschaum, spuma maris, at least 5 varieties, including sponges, algae and corals, halcyon. see 419. **R W H L**
163. Eggs	ova. whites (album), yolks (moel), whole. **B R T W L H Y**
Eglantiere	see 389. **H**
164. (H)Ellebore	eleborum, ellebre, Christmas rose. *Helleborus album and nigrum, Veratrum album.* **R T H Y**
165. Elder	sureau, sambucus, ebulus. juice and a tube of bark slipped off a twig to serve as a cannula. see 406. **B T H**
165a. Elm	slippery elm tree bark. ordinary elm-tree samaras *Ulmus fulva* .**R T**
166. Emeralds	aluminum silicate gemstones, smaragdus, praze, prassium . **W H**
167. Emperor's herb	an umbellifer similar to angelica. *Angelica archangelica.* **W H**
167a. Encaustrum	caustic red ink, or vernis. see 479, 490. *Terminalis vernis.* **T W**
168. Encens	see 188, 316, 463. **R Y**
Endive	see 113, 392. **T H**
Entale	see 152a
168a. Enula	inula, elecampani. see 45, 437. **W H**
169. Epithyme	like cuscuta. see 160. *Cuscuta major and minor.* **W H**
170. Equisetum	asperella, cauda equina, queue equina, horsetail reed, shave grass. *Equisetum arvense.* **T W H**
Ers	see 325. **H**

171. Eruca mustard weed, charlock, rocket-root, sinapus. see 297, 426. *Sinapus avensis.* **R T W**

 Esula see 173, 442. **T W H**

172. Eupatorium agrimony. see 13. **T W**

173. Euphorbia amblete, custos hortis, mardilium, manne, solsequium, esula, titimalle, cataputia. anabulle is the sap. *many varieties of spurges, Euphorbeacea.* **R B T L H Y**

174. Fabaria lovage, water parsnip. see 247, 256. **T H**

175. Faex precipitate at bottom of oil jugs, faex olei. **T W H**

176. Faex cerae beeswax, faex alvearum, eryngium. see 293. **H**

177. Farina de Moulin amidon, far, amylum, farina volatica, mill-dust (fine wheaten flour) also found at bake-ovens, see 21,187,494. **R T W L H**

178. Fava feve, fabba, beans or their stalks, especially *Vicia faba. and Lupinus albus* **R W L H**

179. Feces stercus, topho, tordus; sheep, goat, deer, rats birds, horses etc see 184. **R T W L**

180. Fennel fenoil, marathon. leaves. *Foeniculum vulgare.* **R T L H Y**

181a. Ferns filix. various forms as listed by name

181. Fenugrec aegoceros, buceros, telis. seeds, Greek fennel, ferrugine. seeds usually powdered. see 180. *Trigonella foenum-graecum.* **R B T W L H Y**

 Fermentum see 502. **W H**

182. Fesire white bryony. see 67. **W**

 Fever-few see 454.

 Ficus see 185.

183. Fiel fel, felles, bile (dog, cow, bull, ox, felles avium, colre, choler etc.) see 57. **W L H**

184. Fiente fimus columbinus or equus. pigeon or horse droppings. see 179. **R T L H**

 Figwort see 56.

185. Figs   alos, coctana, citonia. capri ficus is a wild fig. see 84, 260. *Ficus arboris.* **B T W L H**

186. Filipendula   spirea, dropwort. *Spirea filipendula.* **H**

Filonium   philonium, see 320.

Fisticus   see 351. **H**

Flammula   see 120. **L**

Flaura   an herb,variously attributed: a clover, a fumitory. see 122a, 191. **R**

186a. Flos   battitura aeris, aloxan. various films (usually metallic salts) deposited on metals and fluids. see 404, 481, 482, etc. **W L H**

187. Flour   farina, furfur, samich, froment, pigle (coarse-ground). see 177, 395a, 494. **R T W L H**

188. Frankincense   gum resin. see 168, 316. *Boswellia cartorii* . **R B T W L H Y**

189. Fraxinus   bark of ash tree, fiêne, stone-mint. see 264. *Fraxinus excelsior.* **T W H Y**

Frog   see 375

190. Fuchsia   see 334. *Parietaria officianalis.*

190a. Fuligine   soot . **R**

191. Fumeterre   fumitory, gingidium, herba flaura, flama, lady's mantle. see clover *Fumaria officinalis or Gingidium.* **R T L H Y**

192. Fusco   unguentum fuscum, Brown ointment of Nicolas see 306. **R**

193. Galanga   China root. see 276. *Alpinia galanga.* **R T W H**

194. Galbanum   a ferula resin. *Ferula galbaniflua.* **R B T W L H Y**

194a. Galen's Ointment 72, 105, 206, 253, 312, 388, 439, 493. **T L**

Galigan   see 394. **Y**

195. Galles   oak galls.**R B T W L H Y**

196. Gallitricum   salvia, centrum galli, crista galli, oculi christis, sclaria. see 400, 405. **H**

197. Garance   madder root, rubeau, spargula. see 197, 392a, 497. *Galium molugo, G. aparime and Rubia tinctorum..*

198. Garlic   see 43, 278a. **R T W**
     Garyophyla   see 93
199. Gentian   genista. bitter roots of *Gentiana lutea* . **T W L H Y**
     Geranium   see 6, 209.
200. Germander   scordium, polium, chamosdrys, camedrios, yva, ambrosia. see 346, 418. *Teucrium polium and montanum.* **R T W L H**
     Geum   see 93
201. Ginger   zingiber, genevrier, abel. see 14. *Amomum zingiber.* **R B T W L H Y**
202. Girofle   cloves, caryophyllus. see 93. **R Y**
     Git   see 307
203. Glans   acorns (quercus). see 309a. **H**
     Glue   see 368a. **W L**
204. Gluten   gelatin from fish or domestic animals, mucilage, animal collagen, (not from grains). see 124. **R B T W L H**
     Glycyrrhyza   see 246. **H**
     Goat's beard   see 47a.
205. Goatweed   gout-weed, another umbellifer, sometimes Bishops-wort, Agnus caste. *Ammi majus, Aegropodium podagraria* .
     Gold   incinerated or decocted. see 43a. **L**
     Goudron navire   see 304. **Y**
206. Graisse   animal fat—chicken, geese, pork, turtle, etc., pinguedo, sepum, ysopus, bovis, gras, sui, adeps. see 225, 235, 311. Grassede are t he drippings from roasts. **R B T W L H Y**
207. Gramen   seges, couch grass. *Agropyrum repens.* **L H**
     Grana paradisi   see 86, 332. **L H**
208. Grape   uva. leaves and fruit, and skins. raisins, sapa, saramitum, capreoli are the tendrils. see 12. **R T**

208 Grasses and Reeds see 378a, and 386. **R T W H**

209. Gratia dei   geranium. *Gratiola officianalis.* **H**

210. Green Oint.   basically 14 and 273, with supplements by vari-
                           ous authors including 188, 256, 272, 329, 360,
                           424, 459. **R T W L H**

210a. Groseille   currants or gooseberries. see 147 or *Ribes
                           grossularia.* **W H**

211. Gui.   mistletoe. leaves, berries, twigs. *Viscum album.*
                           T W

     Guimauve   see 18, 273

212. Gum Arabic   from acacias. **R T W L H Y**

213. Gummi   sap of cherry, plum, other gums as gumme
                           d'eve, gum evry, Persian gum. see 466. **T W L
                           H**

213a.Gutta Percha   confused with delphinium. see 445.dry gum
                           of *Palaquitum gutta*

214. Gypsum   cockel, selenite, alabaster, plaster of Paris, cal-
                           cium sulfate, gesso. **R T W L**

     Hair   see 111

214a. Halcyon   alcion, caromarina. see 162 **R**

215. Handacote   also septemnerviée. see 428.

     Hawkweed   mouse-ear. see 347

215a. Hawthorne   spina, hazel. fruits and flowers. *Crategus
                           oxyacantha.* **B**

     Hazel   see 134a

215b. Hedera   funis pauperum. see 120. **R H**

216. Hematite   rust, emathitis, pierre sanguinis, lapis san-
                           guinis. see 225, 235, 311. **T W L Y**

     Hemlock   see 116. **T**

     Hemp   see 78. **T**

217. Henbane   jusquiame, hyoscyamus, solathrum, night-
                           shade, belladonna, cassilago, chenille, fabe
                           lupini, hannabane. see 232, 431. **R T W H**

     Henna   see 15.

     Hepatica   see 268.

218. Hericium   sea urchin bristles. ericium, herisson, hircis, lupis iudaici. see 249. **W H**

219. Hermodactyl   digitus hermetis, colchicum and other related tubers. see124a. *Hermodactylus tuberosus.* **R T W L H Y**

Hieracium   see 347.

Hierapicra   see 344c. **W**

Hieromandrea   see 263.

Holly   see 221.

220. Honey   miel, various kinds. hydromel is a mixture with water. see 330. **R B T W L H Y**

Honeysuckle   licium, oculum, caprifolium. see 84, 245a. **R**

Hordeum   see 323. **L H**

Horehound   see 271.

Horse's tail   equisetum. see 170. **W**

221. Houx   bruscus. holly. see 226a. *Riscus aculeatus.* **R T W**

222. Hyacinth   squill, blue-bell, jacinth. see 443. *Hyacinthus nonscriptus.* **T W H**

Hyoscyamus   see 217, 232, 431. **R L H**

223. Hypericon   St. John's Wort. see 287, 501. *Hypericium perforatum* .?**R H**

224. Hypocystus   hypoquistidos. fungus on roots of *Cistinus hypocystus.* **T W L H**

225. Hysop humidus   arabic for lanolin. see 206, 235. **T W**

226. Hyssop   herb hasca. *Hyssopus officinalis.* **W H**

Iara   tere, yres. see 228

226a. Ilex   holly. berries, leaves, bark. see 221. *Ilex aquafolium.* **T**

Ink   see 168a, 490.

Inula   enula. see 168a, 437. **W H**

227. Irundinum   iron. see 228a, etc.

228. Iris   yreos, powdered orris root, eris ustis is burnt iris flowers, oil. *Iris germanica et al.(Illyrica is Iris florentina).* **R T W L H**

228a Iron	fer. see 227, 239, 267, 279, 289, 419. **R T L H Y**	
Isis	see 502a. **T**	
Ivy	see 120	
Jacea	see 414. **H**	
Jacinth	see 222	
John	Saint. see 372a, 401a.	
229. Joubarbes	Jove's beard. house leeks, stonecrop, tettesuriz, poireaux, sticado. see 101, 229, 243, 319, 425. *Sempervivum tectorum.* **R T W H Y**	
230. Jujubes	fruit of the trees. *Zizyphus vulgaris and Z. saturna.* **T Y**	
231. Juniper	savine, sabine. needles, cones, oil. see 479. *Juniperus sabina.* **R H**	
232. Jusquiaime	henbane, aconite, marsilium, faba luparia, luparis, chenille, morel, caniculata, dens caballinus, symphoniaca. see 217, 431. *Hyoscyamus albus and niger.* **R T W H**	
Kabiteji	see 259. **W**	
233. Kekenji	winter cherry. *Physalis alkekenji.* **H**	
Knot grass	see 361.	
234. Labdanum	sometimes ladanum or laudanum. resin of cistus trees, especially see 67.	
Lac	see 286. **H**	
234a Lacca	lactea. a red resin from litmus. see 325. *Roccella tinctoria* .	
Lacertus	see 257	
Lactucca	see 245. **L H**	
Lana succida	see 235, 498. **H**	
Lanceola	see 353. **R H**	
235. Lanolin	suint, lana succida, hysop, ysopus, see 206. **W L**	
236. Lapathum	sorrel, rumex, paradella, lappa, burdock see 395. *Lappatum acutum.* **R T W L H Y**	
236a.Lapis lazuli	powdered blue gem, ferrous sulfate. **T W**	

Larkspur	see 445, 213a.. Confused with caput purgum, or Gutta percha.
237. Laterinum	oil of the small fish. **T**
Laudanum	see 234. **L**
238. Lauriers	lorier, baccis lauri. berries, leaves of bay trees. Laurin is oil of bay leaves. *Laurus nobilis.* **R T L H**
239. Laureole	de-barked daphne twig, spurge laurel, medulla milici. *Daphne laureola.* **R W L H**
240. Lavender	*Lavandula stoechas and L. officinalis.* **T W Y**
241. Lead, filings	limailles, minium. **R L**
242. Lead, white	see 253. **R T W L**
243. Leeks	prassium. see 229, 231, 319, 327.
243a. Lentigo	water-moss, probably sphagnum. See 272. *Sphagnum cymbifolium.* **R T H**
244. Lentils	lens, lentes. **R W L H**
Lessive	see 254.
245. Lettuce	laitues, lactuca, lettue. *Lactuca sativa; Lactuca agresta* i is wild lettuce (escarolle, endive). **R T L**
Levisticus	see 247. **R**
245a. Licium	honeysuckle. See 84. **R**
246. Licorice	liquoritia, herb reglisse. see 381. *Glycyrrhiza glabra* . **T W L H**
247. Ligusticum	levisticus, lovage. see 174, 256, 430. *Ligusticum levisticum.* **L H**
248. Lily	lis, arcus daemoniacus, crinon. usually oil of bulbs and leaves. *Lilium candidum et al.* Lily often included iris, narcissus and gladiolus. **R B T L H**
248a. Lily of the Valley	mayblossom. *Convallaria majdis.* **T**
249. Limacons	limax, limazun. snails with shells. **R T**
Limailles	see 241, 289, 419. **R T H Y**
250. Limes	limo. limes, lemons. see 119. *Citrus limonum.* **H**

251. Lime (stone)   chaux vive, calx, creta, chauz. fresh lime, powdered, used in cylotrum. **R B T W L H Y**

252. Lin   linois, semence, semen lini, flax seeds and oil or meal. *Linum usitatissimum.*. **R B T L H Y**

Linaria   see 420. **R Y**

253. Litharge litargerie, yellow lead oxide. see 242. for litharge nutritum (spumie argentum) see 441. **R T W L H Y**

254. Lixivium   aqua cineris, lessive, lye, see 83. **B T W L H Y**

Lizard   see 257, 446. **R B T**

255. Lolium   panicium, zizania. darnel grass. *Lolium temulentum and perenne.* **R T H**

256. Lovage   see 174, 247. Black lovage is *Smyrnum dusatrum*, "Alexander's Medicine". **T L**

257. Lucertoli   lacertus. lizard. see 446. **B L**

257a. Lucius magna   the broche fish, Esox lucius. **W**

258. Lumbrici   ges entera. earthworms (or maggots). see 499. **R L H**

258a. Lungwort   palam Marina. see 400 *Pulmonaria officinalis.* **R**

259. Lupin   kabitegi, fava, flowers of faba lupina, usually powdered. see 178 *Lupinus album.* **R T W H**

260. Lycium   licium. made from 84. see 185. **W H**

Lye   aqua cineris. see 83, 254. **H**

261. Mace   myristica. see 50, 295. **W H Y**

Madder   see 197, 392a, 474.

Maiden hair   see 7, 363.

Malum punicum see 364. **H**

262. Malum terrae   cyclamen, malot, earth-nut, etc. see 33, 114. **R L H**

Malva   see 18, 273. **BH**

263. Mandragora   mandrake, belladonna. Hieromandrea is a potion based on mandragora. *Mandragora officinarium.* **R T L H Y**

264. Manna   tamarix, ash-tree. see 453. **T H H**

265. Manne   euphorbia, esula resin. see 173. **Y**
266. Manuchriston   like diamargariton, with added honey. **W**
     Marathrum   see 413
266a. Marble   powdered. **L**
267. Marcassita   iron pyrites (sulfites). **T H**
268. Marchantia   liver wort, hepatica. *Marchantia polymorphia and M. conica.* **T L**
269. Margarita   see 342. **R H**
269a. Marine pumace a coral fish. **T**
270. Marjoram   marjolaine, oregano, hortensa, amoracus, maiorama. sweet marjoram. see 324. *Origanum marjorana and O.vulgare.* **T H Y**
     Marrow   see 275. **R T**
271. Marrubium   maruil neir, samsucus, linoscrofon. horehound. *Marrubium vulgare.* **R B T H**
     Marsilia   clover fern **R**
271a. Martiaton   'soldier's ointment'. 1, 51, 72, 238, 270, 312, 394, 400, 493, 496. **T L**
     Mary   Saint. see 401a.
272. Mastic   resin and oil. Lentisco. *Pistacchia lenticus* . **R W L H Y**
273. Mauve   guimauve, mallow (various), althea, sanaticula, malve, ebiscus malaviscum, cubes, dialthea, diante, mallachee. see 18. *Althea officianalis.* **R B T W L H Y**
     Meats   carnes. see 88, 129, 375. **T L**
274. Medlar   nespole, mespilus, the fruit. *Mespilus germanica.* .**L H**
275. Medulla   moelle, meule, midolle, bone marrow, animals and bones are specified. **B T L H**
     Meerschaum   see 162.
     Mel   also miel. honey. see 220. **R T W L H**
276. Meligalata   galanga. see 193. **W**
277. Melilot   corona regia. sweet clover.*Melilotus leucothea and arvensis.* **T L H**

278. Melissa   sweet balm, calamint. see 72. *Melissa officinalis.*
                        T H Y
279. Mellicrate   pomegranate fruit, or a sweet honey-water bev-
                        erage, melograno. **R**
280. Melon   barecha, citrouilles, pumpkin, melo, citri,
                        pepo, squash. see 48. **R T H**
280a. Memitte   yellow-horn poppy. *Glaucum flavum.* **R T H**
281. Menthastrum   wild mint, aquatic mint, horse mint, sisymbri.
                        Menthastrum sylvestris. **R T H**
282. Mercuriale   linozostis, mercurelle. common weed.
                        Mercurialis annua. **T W H**
283. Mercury   argentum vivum. quick-silver, also flower of sil-
                        ver. **T W H Y**
284. Mesûe's Fetid Pills a laxative containing 11, 19, 79, 125, 220, 228,
                        271, 272, 299, 398, 410, 469.
284a. Mesûe's Oint.   19, 65 (old white), 253, 278, 299, 321, 388 (or
                        300), 411, 496. see153. several different reci-
                        pes were attributed to Mesúe. **R B T L H**
285. Mie a pain   mica panis. bread crumbs. see 65. **L**
286. Milk   mother's is lactus muliebris. sow's milk is lait
                        de scroppha, albugasse is donkey's milk, also
                        goat-milk-whey and cheese-water. **T W L H**
287. Millefuilles   yarrow, St. John's herb. *Achillea millefolium, Hy-
                        pericum perforatum et al.* **B T H**
288. Millet   milium, granum. *Panicum miliaceum.* **T**
     Minium   see 241.
288a. Mint   menthe. see 72, 281, 367. **R T H**
     Mistletoe   see 211.
288a. Mithradates   penny cress. *Thrapsus arvense.* **T**
289. Molo molendini   stercus irundini, cimolia, molybdenum. bits
                        of iron or powder from mill grind-stones. see
                        228a. **R T L H Y**
290. Money wart   wood pimpernel, serpentaria, nummularia.
                        See 348. *Lysimachus nummularia.* **Y**
     Morel   see 232, 431. **H Y**

291. Moschus	deer musk. *Moschus moschifer.* **R H**
291a. Moss	muscus, musceline, muscus aquae, sphagnum, etc. see 296. *Sphagnum cymbifolium and Usnea barbata.* **T H**
291b. Moss Ointment	27, 29, 35, 51, 72, 128, 180, 201, 226, 238, 270, 271a, 290a, 309 (oil), 367, 396, 411. **T**
292. Mourons	scarlet pimpernel. see 348.
293. Mu	beeswax. see 176. **W H**
294. Mulberries	mûres, mora, omorusia. see 155, 317a. *Morus nigra.* **L H**
Mullein	see 395.
295. Mummy	momie, mumie, flecks of desiccated cadavers collected from tombs and catacombs. **R B W L**
Muriate of soda	see 404.
Musa	see 393.
295. Muscade	nutmeg, muscat. see 50, 308. **W H Y**
296. Muscus arboris	treemoss, lichen. see 291a. *Usnea barbata.*
Mushrooms	see 11
Musk	see 96, 291, 446. **R T W**
297. Mustard	see 426. *Synapus alba* .**R B T W L H Y**
279a. Mustard Garlic	*Sysimbrium allaria.* **R**
298. Myrobalans	Indian, or yellow. unripe are chebules. emblicus, belliricus. *Myrobalans indica.* **T W L H**
299. Myrrh	mirre, musa, smyrna, resins of commiphora plants. *Balsamodendron myrra.* **R B T W L H Y**
300. Myrtle	seeds, leaves, berries, oil, wood, water. *Myrtis communis.* **R B T W L H Y**
301. Narcissus	daffodils, affodil, asphodel. *Narcissus pseudo-narcissus.* **R B T L H**
302. Nard	spikenard, spic, and oil. see 437, 475. *Valeriana jatamansi and Nardostachys jatamansi.* **R B T W L H Y**
303. Nasturtium	cresson, water-cress, senationes, garden crew. *Nasturtium officinalis.* **B T W H**

304. Navale   goudron de navire, ship tar. see 352, 455. **R B T W**

   Nenufar   farfar. see 491. **L H**

   Nespole   see 274. **H**

305. Nettles   ortie, califex ignita, castrangula, millemorbia. seeds. see 326. *Urtica urens.* **T L H**

306. Nicolas' Ointment see 365. Sometimes confused with Ung. Fuscum (Brown Roman coriander, ciminum, gith. *Nigella sativa.* **B T W H**

   Nightshade   see 217. **T**

   Nitre nitrum. see 402. **R W H**

   Nummulare   see 220. **Y**

308. Nutmeg   muscade, nux muscata, noiz muscate, centrum galle. *Myristica fragrans.* **R L H Y**

309. Nux   meats shells and oils of nuts. chestnuts are castana, hazel nuts are avellanum, nual is walnut, brou is walnut shells. **R T W L H Y**

   Oak fern   see 362

309a Oak tree   quercus, robur, chene. tan bark is cortex stypticus. **W L H**

310. Oats   avoine, aegilope. *Avena sativa.* **T L H**

311. Oesypus   Ysopus, lanolin. see 206, 235. **T W L H**

312. Oil   usually from mature olives, whereas onfacium (318) was made from the thin juice of green olives and was not classed as a real oil. see 317. **R B T W L H Y**

313. Oil of Deben see 53b. from seeds of *Moringa aptera.* **W**

314. Ointments   Apostles', Basilicon, Black, Brown, Diachylon Galen's, Green, Mesües, Martiaton, Moss, Mummy Nicolas', Palm, Populeum, Rhase's Album, Saracenic,William Somer's. **R B T W L H Y**

315. Oleander   shrub. *Nerium oleander.* **T H**

316. Olibanum   thus, frankincense, cortex olibanum. (thus masculinum from Lebanon). see188. **R B T W L H Y**

317. Olives	oil of green or ripe fruits. wood of tree. *Olea sativa.* **R B T W H**
317a. Omorusia	mulberry. see 294. *Morus nigra.* **T**
318. Onfacium	omphacus, infantium. the thin oil of fresh green olives. see 312. **W H Y**
319. Onions	cepa, as distinct from leeks, allium, poirium. see 101, 425. **R T H**
Opirus	see 65
320. Opium	pavot, philonium. seeds and pods of poppy. see 337. *Papaver somniferum.* **R B T L H Y**
321. Opoponax	epoponac, panax. like myrrh a commiphora resin. *Opoponax chironem.* **R T W L H Y**
Orache	see 42.
322. Oranges	fruit or peel, arantium. see 31b, 119. **T**
323. Orges	barley, hordeum. penidium is barley-sugar cake, ptisan and vitis alba are barley broth. *Hordeum vulgare.* **T W L H Y**
324. Origanum	oregano, wild marjoram. see 270. **T W H**
325. Orobe	horobus, bitter vetch, ers, vicia, lacca is the gum. *Ervium ervilia and E.lens.* **L H**
326. Ortie	nettles. see 305. *Urtie pilulifera et al. including Scrofulaferum nodosum.* **T W H Y**
327. Orpiment	orphimentum, auripigmentum. yellow arsenious oxide, used in cylotrum. see 34. **R T W H Y**
Oseille	see 329.
Ossa combusta	see 62
Ossisacara	and ozzizacara, see 330. **B T Y**
Ova	see 163. **H**
328. Ova	formicarum ant eggs. **T L H**
329. Oxalis	rumex, lapathum, wood-sorrel, alleluia, trefoil, oseille. see 395 and 433. **T L H**
330. Oxymel	a honey-vinegar laxative mixture, ozzizacara, osisatum, oxylaxativum. **R T W L Y**
Oyster shells	incinerated and powdered. see 117, 342.

330a. Palm Ointment 32 (red), 105, 121 (silver), 253, 289, 419, 441, 460. **W L H**

330b. Plma marina palam marina., lungwort. see 258a. **R**

331. Palme vert heart of palm or date palm. see 150. **W L H**

Panada see 65. **W**

Panax see 321.

Panicium see 255. **W**

Papaver see 320. **H**

332. Paprika see 86. *Grana paradisi.*

333. Papyrus paper, usually burnt. see 107. **T L**

334. Parietoria pellitory, lichwort, paritarie. *Parietoria erecta and P. diffusa.* **R L H**

334a. Parsnip wild. *Pastinacia sativa.* **T H**

335. Passula agresta. see 12, 478. **W L**

336. Patience wild dock, rumex, oxalis. see 395.

337. Pavot papaver, poppy (seeds). see 320. **Y**

338. Peach persica. fruit, seeds or leaves. *Persica vulgaris or Prunus persica.* **R T H**

339. Pear fruit, flowers, leaves, wine. *Pirus communis.* **T L H**

340. Peas pisum, any type, or beans. see 358.

Pennyroyal see 367

340a. Peony the flower. any of nus Paionia. **R**

341. Peppers piper, serpyllum, various regions. Diatron piperion was made of three kinds of peppers *Polygonum hydropiper.* **W L H**

342. Perles pearls or marguerite flowers. leaves or oyster-pearls. **R T**

343. Persicaria water-pepper, smart weed, cul-rag. *Polygonum varieties and Persicaria hydropiper.* **R H**

344. Persil parsley, selinum is the seed of apium. *Carum petroselinum.* **R T H Y**

Pes corvinus see 142. **W**

344a. Pes leporis Haresfoot clover, sanamunda. see 122a. *Trifolium arvensis.* **T H**

Peter Saint Peter's Herb see 140a, 401a.

344b.Petroleum   oil of. **R**

    Petroselinium   see 29, 344. **L H**

    Pierre de lanternes unidentified. probably crumbled sandstone.
        Y

    Pigle   see 494. **Y**

344c. Pigra   picra, hierapicra and Galen's hierologodion.
        a laxative pill. see, 199, 79, 125, used with or as
        alternative to cochia. Contains 19, 58, 79, 220,
        272, 398, 437. **T W**

345. Pili leporis   see 356. **B T L**

346. Pilium   a germander. see 200. **W**

347. Piloselle   hieracium, hawkweed. *Hieracium pilosella.* **T L
        H Y**

348. Pimpernels   anagallis, scarlet pimpernel, ipia, wood pim-
        pernel is moneywort, a lysimachia. see 292.
        Anagallis arvensis or Stellaria media. **R T W H Y**

349. Pimpinelle   pimprinelle, saxifrage, lesser burnet, anise.
        Sanguisorbe officinalis. **R T H**

350. Pine   stone pine and others. tree bark, seeds etc.
        Pinus pinus. see 134. **H**

    Pinguedo   see 206. **H**

    Piper   serpyllum. see 341. **H**

    Pira   and pyra. see 339. **H**

351. Pistache   fisticus. *Pistacia vera.* **L H**

    Pisum   see 340, 358. **H**

352. Pix   pitch, picula,peize, pix alba and nigra, poix,
        pissa, resin, turbentyne, trementina. see 126,
        304, 359, 360, 379. **R B T W L H**

353. Plantain plantago, many varieties including water-cress, psyllium,
        rib-wort, lanceola, lancelette, policaria,
        quinque nervicium, arnoglossa, waybread, yva.
        see 428. *Plantago psyllium, P. cynops, etc.* **R T W L
        H Y**

354. Plomb brûle	alanauch, plumbum ustum, yellow oxide of lead. see 242, 253. **R W L H Y**
355. Plum	prune, prunella, plums, tree sap (see gummi), seneste, sebeste Damascus, etc. Diaprunum is an electuary of plums. *Prunus domestica*. **T L H Y**
356. Poil de lievre	pili leporis, hare's-beard (Great Mullein). see 457. *Verbascum thapsus*. **R T W H Y**
357. Poireux	garlic. see 43. *Allium porrum*. **W**
358. Pois	pisum, peas of all kinds. *Pisum sativum*. **H**
359. Poix greque	probably hemlock tree resin, see pix. **R W**
360. Poix (noir)	shoe-makers' pitch or wax. **Y**
360a. Polycaria	pulicaria. inula. see 168a. **T**
361. Polygonum	knot grass, corrigiola, cesune, geniculata. *Polygonum aviculare*. **T L H**
362. Polypode	oak fern, beech fern. *Polypodium vulgare or Gymnocorpium dryopteria*. **R T W L H Y**
363. Polytric	beech fern, hair-cap moss, golden maiden hair fern. *Polytrichium juniperium*. **R T W**
363a Poma	Apples, pears, etc. fruit, wood, leaves, bark. **T L**
364. Pomegranate	malum punicum, pomme gernette, fruit, leaves, flowers or bark (ecorce, cortica), mellicrate, psidia (the fruit peel), melograno, wine, water. *Punica granatum*. **R B T W L H Y**
Pomme de terre	see 114. **R**
364a Poplar	aspen. leaves. buds are oculi populi and bourgeons, bacca, aigeros. see 365. *Populus tremuloides*. **T L H Y**
Poppy	see 320. **R B T W L H Y**
365. Populeum Oint.	also populeon (contained poplar tree-buds—bourgeone de peuplier) also called Nicolas' Ointment, one of several recipes included. 44, 49, 217, 263, 336, 348. **R T W L H Y**

365a.Porrum	ptasion, prassium, garlic. see 43. **R**
366. Portulaca	wild and domestic. purslane, chicken-feet, olus fatuum, Herb Robert. see 368. *Lepidum campestre and L.ruderale.* **T L H Y**
367. Pouliot	pulegium, pennyroyal, polial roial, Dragon-tea used mint. *Menthe pulegium.* **R T W Y**
368. Pourpier	purslane. see 366. *Portulaca oleracea.* **H**
Prassium	emerald gems as well as garden leeks. see 166. **R W**
368a. Propolis	bee glue and wax. see 293. **T H**
368b. Prunella	self-heal. *Prunella vulgaris.* **T H**
Prunum	see 355. **H**
Psidia	see 364 (the peel).see 364. **T H**
Psyllium	see 353. **T L H**
Pulegium	see 367. **T W**
Pumace	see 269a.
368c.Pumice	spuma maris. see 162. **T H**
369. Pumpkin	citrouille, zucca. see 48, 280.**H**
Purslane	see 368.
370. Pyrecanthum	lycium. **T H**
371. Pyrethrum	peretrum, pellitory. flowers of fever-few, chry-santhemum. *Anthrum pyrethrum.* **R B T H Y**
Quercus	see 309a.
372. Quince	coing, cotonia, cydonium malum, citonium malum. pulp and seeds. see 123. *Pyrus cydonia.* **T W L H**
372a Ragweed	St. John's wort. *Senecio jacobea.* **T**
373. Raifort	radish, raiz, horse-radish, rapistrum, raphanus, rave. *Cochlearia armoracia, Raphanus sativus and other Raphani.* **R T W L H**
Raisins	uva passa. see 473. **T H**
374. Ramich	an Arabian compound 19, 30 (berries), 93, 195, 299, 308, 318, 264, 407, 433. **H**
375. Rana scortica	frog-meat. **B T**

376. Ranunculus   clematis, pes corvus, crow's feet. see 33, 120, 142. *Flammula jovis.* **H**

377. Rape   a mustard. *Brassica rapa and napus.* **W L H**

378. Rave   turnip or radish. see 373 and 377.

378a. Reeds   canes, marsh grass, canne, panicium, darnel etc. see 386. **R T W L H**

379. Resin   gumma pini. pine pitch rosin. see 352. **R T L H**

380. Realgar   red arsenic ore. see 34 and 327. **B W L H**

381. Reglisse   licorice. see 246. **W**

381a Rhazes' Oint.   Ung. album, contained 17, 77, 105, 163(whites), 253, 388, 493.

382. Rhubarb   *Rhabarbarum of many species.* **W Y**

Rib-wort   see 353.

Robert's Herb   see 366. **Y**

383. Roche   see 20.

Rocket-root   see 171. **T**

384. Rognons   (oil from) castrated testes,—calves, sheep, etc. **T**

Ronces   see 393.

385. Rosat   roset, rosamel, honey with crushed rose petals. **R W Y**

386. Roseau   marsh reeds, canne. see 378a. *Arundo donax* **W.**

387. Rosemary   herb. *Rosemarinus officinalis.* **W**

388. Roses   oleum rosarum, oil of petals. **R W L H Y**

389. Roses   powder of petals or whole flowers including the anthers. Eglantier are wild roses. see 53c. *Rosacea, var. species.* **R T W H**

390. Roses   syrup of petals, see 385. **H**

391. Roses   water of petals, eau roset. **W H Y**

392. Rostrum porcinum endive. see 113. *Cichorium endivia.* **W H**

392a.Rubia   madder. see 197,474, 497 *Rubia tinctoris.* **T H**

393. Rubis   blackberry, bramble, framboisier, rovo. ronces rouge are unripe. *Ronces nemorosus et al.* **R T H Y**

394. Rue	herb ruta, moly, galigan. oil. *Ruta angustifolia and R. graveolans. A. montana.* **R T W H Y**
395. Rumex	patience, sorrel, oxalis, lappa, burdoch, dock, acedula, great mullein, shepherd's crook. see 236, 433. *Rumex acetosa et al.* **T W H**
395a. Rye	flour. silligo. *Secale cereale.* **T**
396. Sabina	cypress, or juniper. the resin is sandarac. see 149, 479. **T**
397. Saccharum	see 220, 293.
397a. Safflower	see 91. not 398. *Carhamus tinctorius.*
398. Saffron	safron, colchicum, zafranatis, crocus. see 91 and 219. *Crocus sativus.* **R T W L H Y**
399. Sagapenum	another ferula plant resin. see 429 *Ferula persica.* **R B T Y**
400. Sage	many varieties. herb salvia, sange, lungwort, palma marina, pulmonaria. see 258a, 405. **R T L H Y**
401. Sagimen	aphroniton, spuma nitri. precipitate of potassium nitrate. **H**
401a Saints' Plants	herbs, plants, worts, etc. Saint Bennett's, see 116. Saint John's, see 13, 35,172, 223, 287 Saint Mary's, see 49. Saint Peter's, see 140a.
Sal armoniac	see 424. **W L H Y**
Sal baurachi	see 63, 402. **W**
402. Sal de nitre	nitrum, bourrach, borax, nitre, saltpeter. **R W L H**
402a Salex	salix. see 495 **H.**
403. Saliva	spittle. **R T L**
403a Salsola	marsh samphire, glass-wort. see 140a, 487, 501
404. Salt,	sal. common or rock, sel gemma, brine, aloxan (brine 'flower'), muriate of soda. **R B T L H Y**
405. Salvia	sage (many varieties), centrum galli, also darnel, cockle, clary, ieble, salge-damasche, salge-savage. see 196, 400. *Salvia officinalis.* **R H**

406. Sambucus	elder tree, sureau, seu, ebulus. see 165. *Sambucus nigra*. **R L H**
406a. Samphire	saphira, sanguinaria, glass-wort, marine crest. see 140a, 400a, 487, 501.**T H**
407. Sandalwood	sandalus. *Santalum album and rubium*. **R T W L H**
Sanamunda	see 25, 93. **H**
Sandarac	the resin. see 396. **H**
408. Sang dragon	sang de dragunt, sedge. resin of *Calamus draco*. **R B T W H Y**
Sanguinaria	see 140a, 406a, 487, 501. **H**
409. Sanguis	blood: goat, sheep, deer, tortoise, bat, frog, snake, ox, dove hare, menstrual etc. **B T H**
Sapa	see 208, and sappa michum, a syrup with honey. **R**
409a. Saracenic ointment	102, 105, 173, 206, 242, 242, 286, 368c. **R T**
410. Sarcocolla	argemone. resin of *Pinea mucronata or Astragalus fasciculoformis*. **R B T W L H Y**
411. Saturieia	herb savory. *Satureia hortensis*. **T H**
411a. Satyrion	an aphrodysiac orchid. see 472. *Satyrion hircinum*. **W**
412. Savon	sapo, soapwort, saponaria, burith. soap. see 430d. **R T L H**
413. Saxifrage	marathrum. flowers or leaves. see 27, 349. **T H**
414. Scabieuse	devil's bit, scabious, jacea, knautia arvensis, morsus diabole. *Centurea scabiosa*. **R T L H**
415. Scalonée	bulbus, scallions, onions. see 319. **W**
416. Scammony	bindweed, convolvulus, anabula, diagridum. *Scammonaciae, several varieties*. **T W L H**
Scariola	see 113. **T H**
416a. Schoenanthum	palea camelorum, juncus. see 444. **H**
417. Scoloprendre	ceterach, hart's-tongue fern, cow-tongue, bugloss, blue weed. see 69. **W**
418. Scordium	wood sage, a germander. see 200. *Eucrium scordium*. **W**

418a. Scorpion	incinerated. **L**
419. Scorie de fer	ferrugo, iron filings and rust, merda ferri and cimolea, limailles. see 216.**W**
420. Scrofularia	pennywort, centumcellie, toad-flax, umbilicus venus, linaria. Many varieties of *Scrofularaciae nodosum, aquativca, etc. Linaria vulgaris.* **R T L Y**
421. Sebestes	sebesten, cordia myra. see 355. **T Y**
422. Sedge	see 74, 408, 434, 444. **L**
422a. Sedum	stonecrop. See 446b. **R**
423. Seeds	common seeds, including lettuce, endive, purslain, chicory, melons. see 123a. **R T W**
424. Sel armoniac	sal ammoniac, ammonium chlorhydrate, commonly called"arsenic". **B W L Y**
Selinum	see 29, 344. **L**
425. Sempervivum	crassula minor, house leek, leeks, joubarbe, sticado. see 229. **R T W L**
426. Senape	synapus, senevé, mustard. see 297. **R B T W L**
Senecio	also senacio. groundsel see 102. **T**
427. Senna	many cassia varieties. see 94. *Cassia fistula* is a potent laxative. **T W**
428. Septemnerviée	handacotte, centinervia, ribwort, quinquenervia, possibly tormentil or septfoil. see 353. **R T**
429. Serapinas	serapias, sarapinas, sagapenum. see 37, 399. *Ferula persica.* **R W L Y**
430. Sesali	lovage, white gentian. see 247. *Laerpitum siler.* **W**
Shepherd's Crook see 395.	
Sifula	sider, aneth . see 26b.
430a. Silex	flint. **Y**
Siligo	rye. see 187 (white). **T W L H**
430b. Silver	argentum. flos, ashes. **L**
Sisymbro	horse-mint, menthastrum. See 281. **R**

430c. Skin	cow and sheep, for making collagen, parchment, pellis, solea. see 204, 431. **R W**
430d Soap	gallic soap, etc.see 412.
Snails	see 249. **T**
Snake-root	serpentaria. see 33, 500.
Soapwort	see 412. **R**
Socotrin	succatrensis.see 19. **W**
431. Solathrum	nightshade, henbane, solanum, morele, camel, mors canis. see 217, 232.*Solanum nigrum et al.* **R T L H**
431a. Solea	leather, soglia. See 124, 204, 368a, 430c. **R**
431b. Soot	fuligine **R**
432. Sorba	cormes. fruits of the mountain ash. see 189, 264. *Sorbus domestica, and Sorbus ancuparia.* **T L H**
433. Sorrel	oxalis, oseille, rumex, lapathum. see 329, 395. **T**
434. Souchet	a sedge, see 5, 74, 75, 408, 422, 444.
435. Spathula foetida	stinking iris. *Iris foetidissima.* **R T H**
436. Spelt	epeautre, hard wheat. see 21, etc. **W**
436a. Sperm	goat. **T**
437. Spic	spikenard, nard. see 302, 475.*Valeriana officinalis, Inula conyza et al* . **B T W L H Y**
Spina	see 215a. **B**
438. Spider web	toile d'araignée, tela aranea. cobweb. **B H**
438a. Spig	any lichen, especially *Lichen gyratis.* **W**
438n. Spleen-wort	a scaly fern. *Asplenum ceterach.* **T**
439. Spode	zinc oxide, tuthie, pompholyx, cathimia. see 121. **W L**
440. Spodium	calcined arrowroot. *Maranta arundinacia.* **L H**
Sponge	see 117. **R T H**
441. Spuma d'argent	écume d'argent, flower of silver. see 253. **R T W**
441a Spuma maris	magnesium silicate, meerschaum. see 162. **W L H**

442. Spurge	resin of a euphorbium. see 173. *Euphorbia lathyris.* **R T L**
442a Squid	os sepiae, seiche, sepia. burnt bone. see 62. **T H**
443. Squill	wild hyacinth. see 222. *Scilla maritima.* **R T L H**
444. Squinanthus	sinancie, another calamus, schoenanthum. see 5, 74, 75, 408, 416a 422, 434. *Andropogon schoenanthus.* **R T W L**
444a.Stag's horn	any fern of genus *Platycerum.* **T**
445. Staphisagre	larkspur, delphinium, cheif d'espurge, polycaria, pes alanda, jonquarola. *Delphinium staphisagre or inula policaria.* **R T W H Y**
445a. Stellaria	chick-weed. morsus gallinae. *Stellaria media.* **H**
446. Stellion	gaulus, a musk-like excrement of lizards. see 257.**W**
Stercus	see 179. **W**
Sticado	see 229, 446a. also *Stoechas citrinus, Graphalum stoechas.*
Stoechas	many varieties. see sticado and 240. also *Stoechas arabica.* **W H**
446b.Stonecrop	vermiculartis.*Sedum acre.* **R**
Styptica	see 309a.
447. Styrax (storax)	assefan, liquid amber, cozembrun, calamite is inferior grade storax. see 36. *Liquidambar orientale (a tree).* **R B T W L H**
447a Sudor	sweat, animal or human. **R**
448. Sugar	alun de sucre, zuccharum, sugar candy, penedis is a droplet of sugar, sugar of violets or roses etc. **R B T W L H**
Sureau	see 165. **Y**
449. Sumach	the posonous toxicodendron. *Rhus coriaria* as well as non-poisonous *R. aromaticum.* **B T L**
450. Sulfur	zolfo. often stated as 'live', being fresh from the mine. **R T L H**

450a. Swallow-wort   milk-weed. *Cynanthum vincitoxicum.* **T**

450b. Sycamore   plane tree. sap. *Platanus var.species.* **Y**

451. Talpa   the mole. **H**

452. Tamarind   tamarind fruit. *Tamarindus indica.* **T W L Y**

453. Tamariscus   sap of manna, ash tree. see 264. *Fraxinus ornus, Mysicaria germanica.* **R T W H**

454. Tansy   athanasia, tanasie. *Tanacetum vulgare.* **T H Y**

455. Tar   naval, Greek. see 304, 359. **R B T H**

Tarragon   see 161a.

456. Tartar   potassium bitartrate from wine lees. **R T L H Y**

457. Tassus Barbatus   tassebarbatus. great mullein (bouillon). see 356. *Verbascum t hapsus.* **R T W H**

458. Teazle   chardun thistle, dipsacus, cardo. see 100, 102, 159. **T**

Tenacetum   see 454

459. Terebinth   also olibanum, xylobalsamum. closely related to mastic. alkitron is a distillate. see 272. also *Pistacia terebinthus* . **R W L H Y**

Terpentine   see 352.

460. Terra sigillata   an astringent trochee of baobab fruit, *Adansonia digitata*, or a reddish clay of Lemnos, fashioned like an Egyptian seal. chimolia or cymolea. **R T W L H**

461. Thapsus   tapsie, another scrofularia umbellifer. see 36. *Thapsia villosa and Th. garganilla.* **R T H**

462. Theriac   many formulas through the centuries. The diatesseron variety contained 58, 199, 220 and 238(berries). Recently called treacle. **T L H**

Thistle   see 458 et al.

463. Thus   cortex thuris. a thick frankincense, see 188, 463. *Boswellia thurifera.* **B W L H**

464. Thyme   calamint. *Thymus capitatus.* **T H**

Titimalle   see 173. **R T H**

Tongue   see 69

464a.Tonnina   Mediterranean tuna. **T**

465. Tormentilla   sarsaparilla, quinquefolum, cinqfoil, potentilli, geranium maculatum, cranesbill or doves-foot, pie de colomb, pseudoselinon, callipetalon. *Potentilla reptans.* **T H**

466. Tragacanth   dragacanth *Astragalus gummifer.* **R B T W L**

Tremula   see 364a (quaking aspen). **T**

467. Tribulus   water thistle, water chestnut or Burra Gukaroo. *Tribulus terrestris or T. aqautica.* **H**

Triticum   see 494.

468. Tryphére   an electuary containing truffles and various sweets.

469. Turbith   turpeth, root of *Operculum turpathum.* **B T L**

Turmeric   see146 and 503. **T W L H**

Turpentine   see 352.**R T W L**

470. Tussilage   colt's foot. *Ungula caballina.* **H Y**

471. Tuthie (tutty)   see spode. see 121, 439. **R T L H Y**

Umbellicus venus   cymbalaria. see 136, 420. **R L H**

472. Unguis caprae   goat slipper. see 411a. **H**

472a Urine   animal and human. **B T H**

Urtica   see 305, 326. **H**

Uva   see 208.

473. Uva passa   raisins. **T H**

474. Valania   madder. see197, 392a. *Rubia tinctorium..*

474a. Valdemona   unidentified. **R**

475. Valerian   phu, amatilla, fistra. spikenard. see 302, 437. **T H Y**

476. Venus hair   maidens-hair fern, capillus venus, bed-straw. see 7. *Adiantum capillus veneris.* **T H**

Venus ointment   see 30

477. Verbena   vervaine, hiera botane, verminacula. *Verbena officinalis.* **R T W L H Y**

478. Verjus   agresta, vinum acerbum, a potion from sour grapes or other sour fruits. see 12, 335, 485.

478a. Vermicularis   stone-crop, sedum. see 446b.

Vermis   see 499. **H**

479. Vernis   vernice, juniper tree sap. *Thuia articulata.* sometimes Encaustrum. see 168a. **T H**

480. Vespa   wasp. **H**

481. Vert d'Airain   vert d'araim, ziniar, fleur d'arain, flos aeris, viride aes, bronze flower, same as 482. **R T L H Y**

482. Vert de Gris   copper 'flower', copper acetate, chloride or sulfate. see 106, 481. **R T W L H Y**

483. Vetch   ers, orobe. see 325. **L**

484. Vinegar   acetum, aisil. **R B T W L H Y**

485. Vinum goretum   raw styptic wine. see 12, 478.

486. Violets   oil of or water of many varieties of *Violaria*. **R B T L H**

487. Virgo pastoris   shepherd's purse, another dipsacus, sanguinary, centinodium, passerinus, proserpinaia. see 406a. 501. *D. sylvestris.* **T W L H**

488. Virgo cervi   deer's penis. **H**

489. Viticella   white bryony, vitis. see 67, 120 etc. *Clematis flammula.* **R L H**

490. Vitriol rosa   red iron sulfate, couperose, atrament, chalcantum, colcothar, ink, Roman vitriol. **R T W L H Y**

490a. Water chestnut   *Trapa natans.* **T**

Water cress   see 353. also *Nasturtium officianale* . **R**

491. Water lilies   nenuphar, dardana, fafara. *Nymphea alba.* **T L H**

492. Watermelon   copcomero. fruit. see 280. **R**

492a Water mint   *Mentha aquatica.* **T**

492b Waters   sea, rain. see 286, 300, 364, 391 et al. **H**

493. Wax   white and red (cera alba and rossa), cere, sire. **R B T W L H**

494. Wheat   froment, triticum. pigle is coarsely ground. see 21. **T L**

494a. William Somer's Ointment	white resin (379) and 485. **T L**
Whey	serum. especially goat's. see 286.
495. Willow	salex. withe. tree bark, and flowers *Salix alba and nigra.* **L**
496. Wines	many varieties, named by color, region, potency, acidity, thickness. see 485. **R B T W L H**
Winter seeds	the four cool-weather seeds. 137,144, 280, 492. see 123a. **T**
497. Woad	pastel, the dye. see 392a. *Ivatis tinctoria.*
498. Wool	laine muste, lana succida, unwashed fleece. **R B W**
499. Worms	lumbrici, ver, verm. see 258. **T L**
Wormwood	see 1.
Xylobalsamum	see 459
500. Yari	cuckoopint arum, serpentaria. see 35a. *Arum maculata.*
501. Yarrow	mille feuille, sanguinary. see 223 287. **B**
502. Yeast	fermentum. leaven. **H**
Yerasimum	unidentified laxative. **Y**
Yreos	see 228.
Ysopus	see 206, 225, 311.
502a. Ysis	isis. any lichen of genus *Isidium.* **T**
Yva	gum eve, iva arthretica, a germander. see 353. *Teucrium chamaedrys.* **T**
503. Zedoaria	turmeric. see 146. *Curcuma longa et al* .**H**
Ziniar	see 482.
Zinziber	see 201. **H**
Zizania	see 255
Zucca	pumpkin. see 369 **R**
Zuccharum	see 448. **W**

www.ingramcontent.com/pod-product-compliance
Lightning Source LLC
Chambersburg PA
CBHW020719210526
45160CB00012B/36/J